Anti-Inflammatory Diet Cookbook for Beginners:

170 Secret Simple Recipes to Boost Your Immune System and Drastically Reduce Inflammation!

Table of Contents

Introduction 3

Chapter 1: Why You Might Need the Anti-Inflammatory Diet 8

Chapter 2: Foods That Cause Inflammation 13

Chapter 3: Anti-Inflammatory Diet Shopping List 22

Chapter 4: Mediterranean Diet 35

Chapter 5: DASH Diet 49

Chapter 6: Anti-Inflammatory Breakfast Recipes 55

Chapter 7: Anti-Inflammatory Lunch Recipes 93

Chapter 8: Dinner Recipes 137

Chapter 8: Snack Recipes 179

Chapter 9: Seven-Day Meal Plan 189

Conclusion 192

Introduction

I got started on the anti-inflammatory diet when I looked for a natural way to treat arthritis. I didn't want to take meds since I was more interested in a holistic and all-natural solution.

My doctor suggested that I try different kinds of anti-inflammatory diets. I started with the DASH diet, well because I also had an elevated blood pressure. I later switched to an anti-inflammatory diet that was better suited for my needs.

I have tried hundreds of recipes, some of which were recommended by friends who cared enough to support me in my endeavor. After being on this type of diet for about a year I noticed that my arthritis was greatly alleviated, my blood pressure wasn't skyrocketing, and that I was generally healthier.

It took a little over a year before the weight loss benefits became obvious and visible but I did lose weight safely and moderately. I didn't feel that I was restricted in my food choices and I should say that this was the best diet I have ever tried.

In fact, I have decided to live an anti-inflammatory lifestyle. I no longer crave sweets that much. I still have sweets and maybe a beer or two every once in a while. This diet has allowed me to live a fuller and healthier life.

In this book I have included my favorite recipes as well as information and expert advice on the anti-inflammatory diet that I have learned in my years of experience living this kind of lifestyle. Some of the information that I share here were also furnished to me by fitness trainers and doctors who worked with me as I transitioned into this type of eating plan.

I have also outlined two types of anti-inflammatory diets—the DASH Diet and the Mediterranean Diet—so you can try them as well. Each of these diets has its pros and cons. I have also included meal plans and recipes for them too.

I encourage you to try the meal plan that I have included in this book. I have made the plan easy to follow and the recipes very easy to access.

Remember that this is an introductory book to the anti-inflammatory diet. The tips and strategies provided here have been designed to help those who want to try and maybe transition into this type of eating plan.

I don't make any promises, but I guarantee that this type of eating strategy is very easy to transition into. I have to admit that some people may find it slightly challenging but with tasty and tempting meals, switching to an anti-inflammatory diet shouldn't be that hard.

Once again, I would like to thank you for downloading this book. May you find a bright and easy path to better eating and fuller health.

© Copyright July Anderson 2019 - All rights reserved.

The content contained within this book may not be reproduced, duplicated or transmitted without direct written permission from the author or the publisher.

Under no circumstances will any blame or legal responsibility be held against the publisher, or author, for any damages, reparation, or monetary loss due to the information contained within this book, either directly or indirectly.

Legal Notice:

This book is copyright protected. It is only for personal use. You cannot amend, distribute, sell, use, quote or paraphrase any part, or the content within this book, without the consent of the author or publisher.

Disclaimer Notice:

Please note the information contained within this document is for educational and entertainment purposes only. All effort has been executed to present accurate, up to date, reliable, complete information. No warranties of any kind are declared or implied. Readers acknowledge that the author is not engaging in the rendering of legal, financial, medical or professional advice. The content within this book has been derived from various sources. Please consult a licensed professional before attempting any techniques outlined in this book.

By reading this document, the reader agrees that under no circumstances is the author responsible for any losses, direct or indirect, that are incurred as a result of the use of information contained within this document, including, but not limited to, errors, omissions, or inaccuracies.

Chapter 1: Why You Might Need the Anti-Inflammatory Diet

What is an Inflammation?

What is an inflammation? The word inflammation refers to a swelling in a localized part of the body. The area that is inflamed is usually hot, reddened, and also painful. It can occur in any part of the body where there is an infection or injury.

The aforementioned symptoms are actually for short term inflammation. There is also long-term inflammation (i.e. chronic inflammation) and that is the type of inflammation that drives diseases.

An inflammation is one of the ways your body protects itself. It also helps fight off infections. In most cases, inflammation is good since it is an essential part of the body's natural healing process.

However, just like every good thing in the world, if you get too much of something—even if it is something beneficial—then it can do more harm than good. Too much inflammation—also known as chronic inflammation—is definitely a problematic condition for anyone.

There are also some people who have a type of medical condition where their immune systems aren't actually functioning efficiently. This condition can lead to low level or short-term inflammation, but it can also result in persistent long-term or chronic inflammation.

Chronic inflammation is a condition that can occur when you get infected or catch other types of diseases. It can happen when you have asthma, rheumatoid arthritis, psoriasis, and others conditions as well. Research indicates that chronic inflammation is also a precedent to cancer.

Other than these diseases, medical research also suggests that our dietary choices may also contribute to chronic inflammation. That means, if you are suffering from any form of inflammation it will help you a lot if you change your eating habits.

Yes it is true that taking meds can help. But if you're looking for a long term and natural way to manage and get rid of chronic inflammation, then a better option would be to adopt an anti-inflammatory diet.

Signs of Inflammation

Here are some of the signs that you are experiencing inflammation anywhere in your body:

- Loss of appetite
- Bloating around the abdomen
- Acid reflux
- Achy joints
- Nausea
- Cramping
- Gas
- Diarrhea

If you experience any of these symptoms, then you should check with your doctor. They can help you determine whether you do have inflammation or if the symptoms you are experiencing are for another condition.

The good news is that by simply making dietary changes you can slowly reduce inflammation in your body naturally. It is the slow and steady approach to long term improved health. You can do that by adopting the anti-inflammatory diet.

What is the Anti-Inflammatory Diet?

According to the Arthritis Foundation, there is actually no specific anti-inflammatory diet for any health condition—including arthritis, of course. There are different types of anti-inflammatory diets.

Examples of anti-inflammatory diets are the Mediterranean Diet and Dr. Weil's Diet. These diets are based on ingredients that either promote or reduce inflammation in the body.

Of course, anti-inflammatory diets will include ingredients and foods that help to reduce inflammation. It also prohibits the consumption of inflammation promoting foods. As such you will notice that the main ingredients in the recipes in this book usually are veggies and fruits.

This is because a lot of plant based foods are rich in antioxidants. According to many studies, antioxidants remove free radicals in the body. Free radicals are molecules that can lead to cell damage when they accumulate.

That is the reason why all anti-inflammatory diets include a lot of anti-oxidant rich food. The goal in such diets is to help the body get cleaned up and maintained internally. With this diet you heal your immune system and improve digestion.

Types of Anti-Inflammatory Diet

There are many popular diets today which are anti-inflammatory. Examples of anti-inflammatory diets include the DASH Diet, the Mediterranean Diet, and Dr. Weil's Anti-Inflammatory Diet.

We will go over these diets in the next few chapters.

I don't really recommend a specific type of anti-inflammatory diet since every person will have unique needs. You can of course choose to follow any of these three popular diets mentioned above. You can also create your own anti-inflammatory diet meal plan too, which is what I did.

I was able to make my custom plan with the help of a nutritionist. At least I know that the meals I am eating are a good fit for me.

Chapter 2: Foods That Cause Inflammation

We mentioned earlier in the previous chapter that our eating habits and the foods that we eat may cause inflammation. One of the ways that you can kick start your way into the anti-inflammatory diet is to avoid eating inflammation causing foods.

These foods can be placed in six different categories:

1. High Fructose and Sugary Foods
2. Vegetable Oils (Includes Seed Oils)
3. Excess Alcohol
4. Processed Meat
5. Refined Carbs
6. Artificial Trans Fats

Let's go over the details of each of these items and why they can cause inflammation.

High Fructose and Sugary Foods

On the top of our list of foods that you should avoid are sugary foods and foods that contain a lot of fructose. There are two main culprits in our day to day diet that contribute to inflammation.

The first one is high fructose corn syrup and the other one is table sugar. These are the two main types of sugar that is very common in our modern diet. According to one study, these added sugars actually cause a lot of damage to the body.

According to another study, it is possible to develop breast cancer with a high sucrose diet. Sucrose is another form of sugar. It is also suggested that eating sugary foods can prevent or block the anti-inflammatory effects of omega-3 fatty acids.

Now, fructose and all the other types of sugars that you find naturally in all our foods are not bad or evil per se. They're actually good—they give the body its needed energy. What's bad is taking in too much—which can happen really quickly.

Just drink a large can of Coke and you would have ingested all the sugar that your body needs in one week in just one sitting. But do you stop with one can of soda? Some people drink three sodas or more each day.

High fructose intake has been linked to chronic <u>diseases</u> like cancer, fatty liver disease, diabetes, insulin resistance, obesity, and chronic kidney disease.

Foods that usually have high levels of added sugar include the following:

- Certain types of cereals
- Sweet pastries
- Doughnuts
- Cookies
- Cakes
- Soft drinks
- Chocolates
- Candy
- Fruit juices (sweetened ones)
- Any sugar sweetened drinks

Vegetable Oils (Includes Seed Oils)

The average consumption of veggie oils and seed oils has increased in the 20th century by as much as 130%. Experts see it as a contributor to the growing number of health problems caused by inflammation. Researchers believe that increased consumption of these oils causes inflammation.

These oils contain a lot of omega-6 fatty acids. Even though they are necessary to the human body, they actually increase inflammation when there is more omega-6 compared to omega-3 in the body.

Note that vegetable oils are used in cooking and are ingredients in a lot of processed foods as well. Reduce your intake of veggie oils and seed oils so as to prevent the onset or to reduce inflammation in the body.

Excess Alcohol

It can be argued that moderate alcohol consumption does have some health benefits. That means your occasional couple of drinks every now and then isn't really that bad. However, taking in more alcohol than usual will cause serious health problems including inflammation.

People who have a heavy drinking problem may have the tendency to accumulate bacterial toxins in the body—a condition known as leaky gut syndrome. This condition can lead to organ damage and widespread inflammation.

Processed Meat

Processed meat includes beef jerky, smoked meat, ham, bacon, and sausages. They taste great and some people have made them staples on the dining table. However, studies suggest that these foods have been associated with increased risk of a variety of diseases including colon cancer, stomach cancer, diabetes, and heart disease.

The most common illness connected with processed meat consumption is colon cancer. Researchers suggest that this might be due to the fact that these meats contain a large amount of advanced glycation end products or AGEs. AGEs are formed when meat is combined with other substances and then exposed to high temperatures.

Studies confirm that AGEs cause inflammation in the body. Note that there are many factors that contribute to the development of colon cancer. However, research suggests that the biggest contributing factor is probably the consumption of processed meat and the inflammation that comes with it.

Refined Carbs

Not all carbs are created alike. Some are nice to have and there are those that can be a good part of your diet. The ones that are nice to have aren't exactly necessary—and I'm referring to refined carbohydrates.

Note that not every kind of carb is problematic. You see, since ancient times man has been consuming carbs. It's a fact, but our ancestors ate unprocessed carbs and it contained a lot of fiber, which is good for the body.

What has changed in the last hundred or so years is that we have introduced refined carbs. The idea behind using refined carbs is that the refining process lengthens the shelf life of the carbs that we usually produce.

However, in the process of refinement, the fiber and all the other essential nutrients get stripped off. What we have left are the refined carbohydrates. Sure they have really longer shelf life but they can cause a lot of inflammation, according to studies.

Remember that fiber promotes blood sugar control and it basically makes you feel full. That is why you don't crave for more food when you just had a high fiber diet. Fiber also feeds the good bacteria in your gut, which helps to maintain your overall health.

Why are refined carbs bad for you? Research suggests that the bacteria that are responsible for inflammation in your gut feed off refined carbs. When inflammation becomes chronic due to years of poor eating choices, then inflammation in the gut will become problematic.

Refined carbs also have a high glycemic index (GI) compared to unprocessed carbs. When food has a rather high GI, it can raise your blood sugar a lot faster. Studies suggest that eating too much food that have a high GI may cause chronic obstructive pulmonary disease

Artificial Trans Fats

The unhealthiest fats on the planet are none other than artificial trans fats. These are foods that have partially hydrogenated ingredients. What that means is that hydrogen is added to unsaturated fats. Unsaturated fats usually have a liquid form. By adding hydrogen to them they become more solid which makes them more stable.

If you check the label on certain food packages, these are the ingredients that have the words "partially hydrogenated" and then followed by the ingredient name. Most margarine brands have trans fats. They are added to extend the shelf life.

Note however that there are natural trans fats as well. These are the fats that are produced in the body and they can also be found in meat as well as in dairy products. It is the artificial trans fats that studies point to that increases our risk for diseases and also cause of inflammation.

Artificial trans fats also reduce the amount of good cholesterol (HDL) in the body. Studies also show that they also impair the endothelial cells lining our arteries which increase our risk for heart disease.

Foods that are usually cooked with artificial trans fats include certain types of pastries, cookies, packaged cakes, vegetable shortening, margarine, microwave popcorn, French fries, and other types of fast food.

Foods That You Should Buy

Now that you know the kinds of food that you should avoid if you want to get rid of inflammation, we will go over a shopping list of foods that you should buy and eat. All information on that will be covered in the next chapter.

Chapter 3: Anti-Inflammatory Diet Shopping List

You don't have to clear out your fridge on your first day on an anti-inflammatory diet. The first step is to do an inventory of the food that already have in stock. You should also do an inventory of the entire kitchen and pantry as well.

Some of the food that you may already have in stock could already be anti-inflammatory. What you need to do during this inventory is to identify the food that doesn't follow the standard and you either give them away to charity or just throw them away.

So, how do you know which foods you should keep and which ones should go? You already know the categories of pro-inflammation foods from the previous chapter.

You'll find below a rather comprehensive list of anti-inflammatory foods that might be very helpful. I have also placed them in different categories as well.

Animal Protein
- Eggs
- Sardines
- Grass-fed beef, bison
- Chicken breasts, chicken thighs
- Herring
- Wild salmon
- Mackerel
- Lamb

Veggies
- Asparagus
- Arugula
- Avocados
- Artichokes
- Beets
- Bell peppers (any color or variant)
- Beet greens
- Broccoli
- Bok choy and other Asian greens
- Brussels sprouts
- Broccoli rabe (rapini)
- Cabbage (green and red variants)
- Cauliflower
- Carrots
- Chicory
- Celery
- Chard, (all variants)
- Chives
- Chinese cabbage
- Cucumbers
- Collard greens

- Dandelion greens
- Daikon radishes
- Escarole
- Endive
- Garlic
- Fennel
- Jicama
- Leeks
- Kale (all types)
- Mushrooms
- Lettuce (all types except for iceberg—I just don't like those)
- Mustard greens
- Olives (fresh, not canned)
- Okra
- Radicchio
- Onions
- Pumpkin
- Parsnips
- Radishes
- Radish leaves
- Romaine
- Scallions
- Rhubarb
- Rutabagas
- Sea veggies (nori, dulse, kombu, wakame, kelp)
- Shallots
- Sprouts
- Spinach
- Sweet potatoes
- Squash (all variants like winter and summer varieties)
- Tomatillos
- Tomatoes
- Turnips
- Turnip greens
- Watercress
- Zucchini
- Yams

Fruits

- Apples
- Bananas
- Apricots
- Blood oranges
- Blackberries
- Cantaloupes
- Blueberries
- Coconut
- Cherries
- Currants
- Cranberries
- Dried fruit (no added sugar/sulfur/additives)
- Grapefruit
- Dates
- Goji berries
- Figs (fresh)
- Guava
- Grapes
- Kiwi
- Honeydew melon
- Limes
- Lemons
- Muskmelon
- Mangoes
- Oranges
- Nectarines
- Peaches
- Papayas
- Persimmons
- Pears
- Pineapples
- Watermelon
- Pomegranates
- Plums
- Raisins
- Prunes
- Raspberries
- Tangerines
- Strawberries

Nuts and Seeds

- Almonds
- Chia seeds

- Brazil nuts
- Flaxseeds, ground
- Cashews
- Hemp seeds
- Hazelnuts
- Macadamia nuts
- Nut and seed butters (Brazil, almond, cashew, pumpkin, pecan, walnut, sunflower)
- Pine nuts
- Pecans
- Sesame seeds
- Pumpkin seeds
- Tahini paste
- Sunflower seeds
- Walnuts

Herbs and Spices

- Ancho pepper
- Bay leaves
- Basil
- Cardamom
- Black pepper, freshly ground
- Celery seeds
- Cayenne pepper
- Chili powder
- Chervil
- Chipotle powder
- Chilies, red

- Cinnamon, sticks or ground
- Cilantro
- Coriander (ground)
- Cumin
- Cloves
- Dill
- Curry powder
- Five-spice powder
- Fennel seeds
- Garlic, fresh
- Garam masala
- Gomasio
- Ginger, fresh and ground
- Marjoram
- Lemongrass
- Mustard powder
- Mint
- Mustard seeds
- Oregano
- Nutmeg
- Parsley
- Paprika
- Red pepper flakes (crushed)
- Turmeric
- Rosemary
- Peppercorns, black
- Saffron
- Sage
- Star anise
- Sea salt
- Thyme
- Tarragon

Beans and Legumes
- Chickpeas/garbanzo beans
- Lentils, green and brown
- Peas (snow, green, and sugar snap)

Condiments

- Balsamic vinegar
- Avocado oil
- Chickpea miso paste
- Coconut aminos (soy sauce alternative, gluten-free)
- Cocoa powder, unsweetened
- Coconut meat (fresh)
- Coconut, unsweetened flakes and shredded
- Coconut oil
- Extra-virgin olive oil
- Coconut yogurt
- Flaxseed oil
- Honey, raw
- Hemp oil
- Kimchi
- Horseradish
- Medjool dates
- Low Sodium Vegetable broth (organic)
- Pickles
- Mustard, Dijon or whole grain
- Pure almond extract
- Pure vanilla extract
- Pure maple syrup
- Red wine vinegar
- Raw unfiltered apple cider vinegar
- Sauerkraut

- Tomatoes (in a glass jar or sundried)
- Salsa
- Sriracha sauce or hot sauce
- White wine vinegar

Grains (Gluten-Free)
- Amaranth
- Chickpea pasta
- Brown rice pasta
- Buckwheat
- Teff
- Chickpea spaghetti
- Millet
- Quinoa (white, red)
- Oats, gluten-free rolled and steel-cut
- Sorghum
- Rice (black, wild, brown)

Dairy-Free Milk
- Hemp milk
- Almond milk
- Culinary coconut milk (in BPA-free cans)
- Cashew milk
- Oat milk (only from gluten-free oats)
- Coconut milk

Beverages
- Filtered/Purified water
- Herbal teas (any tea that is good for detoxification)
- Green tea
- Freshly squeezed and pressed green juices

Gluten-Free Baking Flours
- Almond flour
- Coconut flour
- Almond meal
- Gluten-free oat flour
- Chickpea flour (garbanzo bean)

Snacks
- Dark chocolate
- Cocoa

Supplements
- Alpha-Lipoic Acid
- Curcumin extract
- Fish oil extract
- Ginger extract
- Resveratrol
- Spirulina

Drinks and Tonics

If you want to try anti-inflammatory foods for now—let's say you don't know if they will be something that you can handle on a daily basis, here are a few recipes that you can try in a flash.

These recipes are drinks and tonics which are very easy to prepare. They make use of the items found in the shopping list provided above.

Ginger and Parsley Juice

Ginger and parsley are powerful anti-inflammatory ingredients. They aid in digestion and help to reduce pain and soreness that you may feel after a workout.

Ingredients

- 1 to 2 inches of ginger
- 1 large handful of parsley
- 2 to 3 celery stalks
- 2 cups of spinach
- 1 green apple
- 1 small cucumber
- 1 lemon

Instructions

Extract all ingredients using a juicer. Mix the extracts in a glass. Enjoy

Bone Broth Tonic

Bone broth, especially those from chicken, promotes better sleep, better memory, and improves mental function. They contain collagen which is beneficial for joint health.

Ingredients

- 1 gallon of water
- 2 lbs. of chicken bones (preferably from free-range chickens)
- 2 tbsp. apple cider vinegar
- 2 chicken feet
- 1/2 cup parsley
- 1 tsp. peppercorns
- 1 tbsp. sea salt
- 2 carrots
- 2 celery stalks
- 1 onion

Instructions

Note that this process will take a while. Combine all ingredients in 10-quart slow cooker. Simmer everything for 24 hours. Occasionally skim the fat. Remove the slow cooker from the heat.

Allow it to cool slightly. Discard any solids that you can scoop from the liquid. Strain the liquid through a colander and place contents in a bowl. Let the chicken bone stock cool down to room temperature. Finally, cover it and then chill inside your fridge.

Turmeric and Lemon Tonic

This tonic contains ingredients that combat brain degeneration. They are rich in antioxidants that neutralize the effects of free radicals. Of course they also help prevent and reverse chronic inflammation.

Ingredients

- Juice of 1 lemon
- The rind of that lemon
- 1 pinch of cayenne pepper
- 1 tbsp. fresh grated ginger
- 1 tsp. maple syrup

- 1 tbsp. fresh grated turmeric
- 3 cups filtered water

Instructions

Combine all ingredients in a small saucepan. Simmer over medium heat. Be careful since you don't want it to fully boil. Turn off the heat when you see the mixture start to steam. Strain the liquid into serving glasses (I use mugs). Enjoy.

You can store any left overs in the fridge. This tonic has a three day shelf life.

Chapter 4: Mediterranean Diet

The Mediterranean Diet scores pretty high in the dietary inflammatory index (DII)—a tool that researchers have used to measure how inflammatory certain foods are. The DII uses markers of systemic inflammation in the body. It is a very scientific and systematic method for measuring how likely a diet will cause inflammation in the body.

The DII particularly takes note of the presence of the following nutrients:

- Flavones
- Isoflavones
- Beta carotene
- Flavonols
- Omega-3 fatty acids
- Vitamin C

Check the label of the foods that you buy and try to see how much of the above mentioned nutrients are contained in the package. If it contains two or more of these nutrients then you have some kind of idea that it is anti-inflammatory.

Now, the Mediterranean Diet is one of the diets that gets the nod from the DII. This is the diet of the folks who live along the Mediterranean Sea ergo its name.

The people who live in that area and eat this said diet are known for longevity, better health, and reduced incidence of chronic diseases. The diet that they are eating is low in saturated fat, low in sugar, and has very little red meat.

There is actually no specific "Mediterranean Diet" since every country that lies along the Mediterranean has very distinct cuisines. The Italians, Greeks, Spanish, and the French all have different and unique cuisines.

However, all of these cuisines have common denominators. They follow many similar principles when it comes to the choice of ingredients and how the food is cooked.

Pros and Cons of the Mediterranean Diet

Note that Mediterranean Diets are balanced diets—it doesn't matter if you follow the Greek, Italian, etc. style. They follow the same principles of acceptable ranges of fat, carbs, protein, and other nutrients.

Pros

- Diverse foods and flavors
- It isn't highly restrictive
- It is nutritionally sound

Cons

- Ingredients are moderately pricey
- Preparing the dishes will require time and effort

Philosophy of the Mediterranean Diet

I like the Mediterranean Diet because it is non-restrictive. You won't feel that you're being deprived of great tasting food. In fact, some of the food that you may already have in your fridge could be acceptable in the Mediterranean Diet.

Here are some basic guidelines that will help you figure out if you are still within the bounds of this type of diet:

1. You should eat more eggs, herbs and spices, poultry, seafood, healthy fats, olive oil, beans and legumes, low fat dairy, whole grains, nuts, fruits, leafy greens,

vegetables, and also wine (the ideal is a little red wine once in a while).
2. You should be eating less red meat in this diet.
3. You are also required to avoid any kind of refined grains, added sugars, processed food, and any ingredients that you can't pronounce on the label.

Mediterranean Breakfast Recipes

To get you started on this type of diet, here is my list of favorite Mediterranean breakfast recipes. At least you can sample what Mediterranean mornings are like and decide for yourself whether you will want to eat this way all day.

Some of them are packed with protein so you would feel full first thing in the morning. You may think that starting your day with leafy greens is unthinkable but with a little practice you will see how tasty and filling they can be too. On top of that they won't cause a blood sugar crash.

Morning Breakfast Salad Mediterranean Style
(This recipe makes 4 servings.)

Ingredients

- 4 eggs
- 2 cups halved cherry tomatoes and/or heirloom tomatoes cut into wedges
- 10 cups arugula
- 1 cup cooked quinoa
- 1/2 seedless cucumber, chopped
- 1 cup whole natural almonds, chopped
- 1/2 cup mint and dill, chopped
- extra virgin olive oil
- 1 large avocado
- freshly ground black pepper
- 1 lemon
- sea salt

Instructions

Boil a pot of water. Bring the water to a simmer. Lower the eggs into the water and simmer for 6 minutes. After that remove from heat and run cold tap water on the eggs. Peel them when cool. The goal is to make soft-boiled eggs.

Combine tomatoes, arugula, quinoa, and cucumber in a large bowl. Drizzle with olive oil. Season it with salt and pepper. Give it a toss.

Divide your salad into 4 servings. Top each plate/bowl with a piece of avocado and an egg. Squeeze lemon on top. Sprinkle almonds and herbs and do a final drizzle of olive oil.

Poached Eggs and Salmon on Toast

Ingredients

- 2 slices of bread toasted
- 1/4 tsp. freshly squeezed lemon juice
- 1 tbsp. thinly sliced scallions
- 1/2 large avocado smashed
- Pinch of kosher salt and cracked black pepper
- 2 eggs, poached
- 3.5 oz smoked salmon
- Splash of soy sauce (optional)

Instructions

Mix smashed avocado and then add lemon juice and salt. Poach eggs. Toast bread. Spread avocado mixture on both slices of bread and add smoked salmon. Place poached eggs on toasted slices.

Splash some soy sauce and cracked pepper. Garnish with scallions, micro greens. Serve.

Honey Almond Ricotta Spread

This is actually a popular recipe recommended to me by a friend and it is very easy to do.

Ingredients

- 1 cup whole milk ricotta
- 1/4 teaspoon almond extract
- sliced peaches
- 1/2 cup Fisher Sliced Almonds
- extra honey for drizzling
- 1 teaspoons honey
- extra Fisher sliced almonds
- whole grain toast
- zest from an orange, optional

Instructions

Mix almonds, almond extract, and ricotta. Combine well. Sprinkle additional almond bits and then drizzle with some honey. Toast your bread. Apply even layer of honey almond spread on toasted bread. Top with honey, sliced almonds, and peaches.

Mediterranean Egg Cups

This is another popular Mediterranean recipe and it is also very easy to prepare.

Ingredients

- olive oil or coconut oil cooking spray
- 1 1/2 cups chopped mushrooms
- fresh basil leaves
- 10 eggs
- 1/2 tsp. garlic powder
- 2/3 cup plain almond milk
- 1 1/4 tbsp. goat cheese crumbles
- 1 1/2 cups chopped roasted bell peppers
- 1/4 tsp. black pepper
- 1/8 tsp. salt

Instructions

Preheat oven to 350 degrees. Use cooking spray and spray over 12 muffin tins. Whisk eggs, pepper, salt, garlic powder, and almond milk until mixture is blended well. Add roasted bell peppers and mushrooms.

Bake for 25 minutes. Remove from oven. Allow them to cool for 10 minutes. Serve with goat cheese and torn fresh basil.

Baked Eggs with Feta and Avocado

This is a delicious low carb breakfast option.

Ingredients

- 2 tbsps. crumbled Feta Cheese
- 4 eggs
- olive oil
- 1 avocado
- salt
- fresh-ground black pepper

Instructions

Preheat oven to 400 degrees. Break eggs into individual ramekins. Place gratin dishes on cookie sheet. Heat them for 10 minutes. Peel avocado and cut each half into 6 slices. Remove gratin dishes and spray with olive oil.

Arrange avocado in gratin dishes with two pieces of egg. Sprinkle with crumbled Feta. Season them to taste. Bake for 12 minutes. Serve while hot.

Mediterranean Breakfast Sandwich with Egg and Roasted Tomatoes

This is a home grown recipe that has been passed on for generations.

Ingredients

1 teaspoon butter

1/4 cup egg whites

Salt and pepper to taste

- 1 tablespoon pesto
- 1 teaspoon chopped fresh herbs such as parsley, basil, rosemary
- 1/2 cup roasted tomatoes
- 1 whole grain seeded ciabatta roll
- 1 tablespoon extra-virgin olive oil
- 1–2 slices muenster cheese (or provolone cheese if you like)
- Kosher salt and black pepper to taste

Instructions

Melt butter on non-stick skillet. Pour egg whites. Season with salt and pepper. Sprinkle fresh herbs. Cook for 3 minutes. Remember to flip once.

Toast bread. Spread pesto on bread. Place egg on bottom half of the toasted slices. Roll and fold egg as needed. Add roasted tomatoes. Top with the other slice of toasted bread.

Instructions for roasted tomatoes

Preheat oven to 400 degrees. Slice tomatoes lengthwise and place on baking sheet. Drizzle with olive oil. Roast for 20 minutes. You know when they're done when the skins look wrinkled.

Greek Yogurt Pancakes

Ingredients

- 1 1/4 cup all-purpose flour
- 2 teaspoons baking powder
- 1/4 teaspoon salt
- 1/4 cup sugar
- 1/2 cup blueberries optional
- 1 teaspoon baking soda

- 3 eggs
- 3 tablespoons butter unsalted, melted
- 1/2 cup milk
- 1 1/2 cups Greek yogurt plain, non-fat

Instructions

Whisk salt, flour, baking soda, and baking powder in one bowl. In a separate bowl, whisk eggs, sugar, Greek yogurt, and butter. Add milk and mix until smooth.

Add Greek yogurt to mixture. Let batter sit for 20 minutes.

Heat the pancake griddle. Brush the griddle with butter. Pour the batter in 1/4 cup batches. Cook until the bubbles form on top. Lift corners of each pancake to check that it's golden browned. Flip pancake and other side. Remove from griddle.

Top each pancake with mixed berries and a scoop of Greek yogurt. Serve and enjoy.

Quinoa and Feta Egg Muffins

Ingredients

- 2 cups baby spinach finely chopped
- 1 cup chopped or sliced tomatoes
- 1/2 cup finely chopped onion
- 1 cup crumbled feta cheese
- 1 tablespoon chopped fresh oregano
- 1/2 cup chopped and pitted kalamata olives
- 8 eggs
- 2 teaspoons high oleic sunflower oil
- 1/4 teaspoon salt
- 1 cup cooked quinoa

Instructions

Pre-heat the oven to 350 degrees. Arrange 12 silicone muffin tins on baking sheet, grease them, and set them aside.

Chop vegetables and heat in skillet. Add onions and vegetable oil. Sauté the veggies for 2 minutes. Add tomatoes. Sauté everything for another minute. Add spinach and sauté 1 minute. Turn off heat. Mix in oregano and olives. Set mixture aside.

Blend eggs until well combined. Pour into a mixing bowl. Add feta cheese, quinoa, and veggie mixture. Add salt to taste. Mix everything until well combined.

Pour mixture into muffin tins. Bake for 30 minutes until eggs are golden brown. Take them out of oven and cool for 5 minutes. You can serve warm or chill them first and then eat them cold. You can even microwave the next day if there are leftovers.

Chapter 5: DASH Diet

DASH is short for Dietary Approaches to Stop Hypertension (DASH). It's actually more of an eating plan rather than actual diet in the modern sense of the word. Just like the Mediterranean Diet, this diet also emphasizes the consumption of food that is rich in calcium, magnesium, and potassium.

These are actually the very same nutrients that can help lower blood pressure. Just like other anti-inflammatory diets, the DASH diet includes a lot of the same fruits and veggies.

You will also be required to eat low fat dairy products, nuts, poultry, fish, and whole grains. One of the reasons why it has become really popular is the fact that is a balanced diet and it is not that restrictive.

It limits the consumption of sugary beverages, sweets, and red meats. Yes, you may these foods but you will only get them on your plate from time to time.

Unique Features of the DASH Diet

What makes the DASH Diet unique is in its emphasis on consuming less salt. Remember that the goal of this diet is to help the person better manage his or her blood pressure. There are actually 2 types of DASH Diets—the standard DASH Diet and the Lower Sodium DASH Diet.

- **Standard DASH Diet**: you are allowed to consume up to 2,300 mg of sodium each day.
- **Lower Sodium DASH Diet**: You can only consume up to 1,500 mg of sodium each day.

Note that in the typical modern diet today you usually consume up to 3,400 mg of sodium and higher.

How to cut back on sodium intake? Here are a few tips:

- Buy foods that are labeled as "no salt added"
- Rinse canned food so as to remove the salt content
- Don't add salt to hot cereal, pasta, and rice
- Use sodium free spices

Here are other unique features of this diet compared to other anti-inflammatory diets:

- Grains: 6 to 8 servings a day
- Vegetables: 4 to 5 servings a day
- Fruits: 4 to 5 servings a day
- Dairy: 2 to 3 servings a day
- Lean meat: 6 one-ounce servings or less each day
- Legumes, nuts, and seeds: 4 to 5 servings a week
- Sweets: 5 servings a week or less
- Fats and oils: 2 to 3 servings a day

Sample 3-Day DASH Diet Meal Plan

The following is a sample 3 day DASH Diet meal plan that you can try. You can use it to try and gauge if this type of diet is for you.

Day 1

Breakfast

- 1 banana
- 1 cup fat-free milk
- 1 cup old-fashioned cooked oatmeal
- 1 teaspoon trans-free margarine
- 1 slice whole-wheat toast

Lunch

- 1 cup fat-free milk
- Tuna salad
- 8 Melba toast crackers

Dinner

- Beef and vegetable kebab
- Cran-raspberry spritzer
- 1 cup cooked wild rice
- 1 cup pineapple chunks
- 1/3 cup pecans

Day 2

Breakfast

- Herbal tea
- 1 teaspoon trans-free margarine
- 1 cup fresh mixed fruits
- 1 cup fat-free milk
- 1 bran muffin

Lunch

- Curried chicken wrap
- 1 cup fat-free milk
- 1/2 cup raw baby carrots

Dinner

- 1 cup cooked whole-wheat spaghetti
- 1 teaspoon olive oil
- 1 tablespoon low-fat Caesar dressing
- 1 nectarine
- 1 small whole-wheat roll
- 2 cups mixed salad greens
- Sparkling water

Day 3

Breakfast

- Decaffeinated coffee
- 1 store-bought whole-wheat bagel
- 1 cup fat-free milk
- 1 medium orange

Lunch

- 12 reduced-sodium wheat crackers
- Spinach salad
- 1 cup fat-free milk

Dinner

- Herb-crusted baked cod
- 1 small sourdough roll
- Herbal iced tea
- 1/2 cup brown rice pilaf with vegetables
- 1 cup fresh berries with chopped mint
- 1/2 cup fresh green beans, steamed
- 2 teaspoons olive oil

In the next chapters we will go over my recommended anti-inflammatory breakfast, lunch, and dinner recipes. I'll throw in a few snacks as well.

Chapter 6: Anti-Inflammatory Breakfast Recipes

#1 Scrambled Eggs with Turmeric
Serves: 1

Ingredients:

- 2 kale leaves (shredded)
- 2 radishes (grated)
- 2 eggs (pastured)
- 2 tablespoons coconut oil
- 1 tablespoon turmeric
- 1 small clove garlic (minced)
- 1 pinch cayenne pepper
- clover and radish sprouts (for topping)

Instructions:

- In a pan over medium heat, put in the coconut oil. Sautee the garlic.
- Crack the eggs into the pan. Stir to cook the eggs until they are scrambled.
- Before the scrambled eggs are cooked thoroughly, put in the kale, cayenne, and turmeric. Stir.
- Transfer onto a plate. Top with the sprouts and grated radishes. Serve.

#2 Chia Seed and Milk Pudding

Serves: 4 glasses

Ingredients:

- 4 cups coconut milk (full-fat)
- 1 cup mixed berries (fresh, for garnishing)
- 3/4 cup coconut yogurt (for topping)
- 1/2 cup chia seeds
- 1/4 cup coconut chips (toasted, for garnishing)
- 3 tablespoons honey
- 1 teaspoon turmeric (ground)
- 1 teaspoon vanilla extract
- 1/2 teaspoon ginger (ground)
- 1/2 teaspoon cinnamon (ground)

Instructions:

- In a mixing bowl, put together the ginger, cinnamon, turmeric, vanilla extract, honey, and coconut milk. Mix them well until the mixture turns yellowish in color.
- Put in the chia seeds into the mixture. Mix them well. Leave the mixture undisturbed for about 5 minutes. After 5 minutes, stir the mixture one more time.
- Cover the mixture. Put it in the fridge overnight or at least 6 hours to chill. The

chia seeds will become plump thus giving a thick pudding-like texture.
- Portion the pudding into 4 glasses. Top each glass of pudding with coconut yogurt, coconut chips, and mixed berries. Serve.

#3 Protein-Rich Turmeric Donuts

Serves: 8 mini donuts

Ingredients:

- 7 Medjool dates (pitted)
- 1 1/2 cups cashews (raw)
- 1/4 cup coconut (shredded)
- 1/4 cup dark chocolate (for topping)
- 1 tablespoon vanilla protein powder
- 2 teaspoons maple syrup
- 1 teaspoon turmeric powder
- 1/4 teaspoon vanilla essence

Instructions:

- In a food processor, put in all the ingredients except for the dark chocolate. Blend on high setting until it becomes smooth and sticky dough.
- Portion the dough into 8 balls. Press each ball firmly into a donut mold.

- Cover the mold. Put the donuts in the freezer for about 30 minutes.
- In a saucepan over medium heat, put in a cup of water. Bring the water to a boil.
- In a smaller saucepan, put in the dark chocolate. Place the smaller saucepan on top of the saucepan with boiling water. Stir the chocolate until it is melted.
- Take the donuts out from the freezer. Glaze the donuts with the melted chocolate. Serve.

#4 Nutty Choco-Nana Pancakes
Serves: 10 pancakes

Ingredients:

Sauce:

- 4 tablespoons cacao powder (raw)
- 1/4 cup coconut oil

Pancakes:

- 2 bananas (ripe)
- 2 eggs (large)
- 2 tablespoons creamy almond butter
- 2 tablespoons cacao powder (raw)
- 1/8 teaspoon salt

- 1 teaspoon pure vanilla extract
- Coconut oil (for greasing)

Instructions:

Sauce:

- In a saucepan over low heat, put in the coconut oil. Mix well the cacao powder into the oil. Take out from the heat. Set aside.

Pancakes:

- Pre-heat a skillet over low heat. Put in a tablespoon of coconut oil to grease the skillet.
- In a food processor, put in all the ingredients for the pancake. Pulse the mixture on high setting until the batter becomes smooth.
- Pour about 1/4 cup of the batter onto the pre-heated skillet to make one pancake. Cook each pancake for 5 minutes on one side. Flip the pancake carefully to the other side. Cook the other side for 2 minutes more. Keep doing this step until there is no more batter left.
- Serve the pancakes with the sauce on the side or on top.

#5 Cranberry and Sweet Potato Bars

Serves: 16 bars

Ingredients:

- 1 1/2 cups sweet potato purée
- 1 cup almond meal
- 1 cup cranberries (fresh)
- 1/4 cup water
- 1/3 cup coconut flour
- 2 eggs
- 2 tablespoons maple syrup
- 2 tablespoons coconut oil (melted)
- 1 1/2 teaspoon baking soda

Instructions:

- Pre-heat your oven to 350 degrees Fahrenheit.
- In a mixing bowl, put in the water, sweet potato puree, maple syrup, eggs, and melted coconut oil. Mix them very well.
- In another mixing bowl, sift the coconut flour, almond meal, and baking soda. Mix them very well.
- Put the dry mixture into the liquid mixture. Mix the batter very well.
- Grease a square baking pan (9"). Line it also with parchment paper.

- Put the batter onto the lined pan. Spread the batter evenly using a wet spatula. Press each cranberry on top of the batter.
- Bake for 35 minutes or until cooked through. Slice it into 16 bars after it is completely cooled.

#6 Turmeric Scones

Serves: 6 scones

Ingredients:

- 1 cup almonds (roughly chopped)
- 1 1/3 cup almond flour
- 1/4 cup red palm oil
- 1/4 cup arrowroot flour
- 3 tablespoons maple syrup
- 1 tablespoon coconut flour
- 1 teaspoon vanilla extract
- 1 teaspoon turmeric
- 1/2 teaspoon black pepper
- 1 egg
- Pinch salt

Instructions:

- Pre-heat your oven to 350 degrees Fahrenheit.

- In a mixing bowl, put in all the dry ingredients. Fluff them using a fork.
- In another mixing bowl, put in the vanilla extract, maple syrup, red palm oil, and egg. Whisk them together. Pour the mixture into the dry mixture. Mix them well to form a dough. Flatten the dough into an inch thick round shape form just like pizza dough. Slice the dough into 6 scones.
- Arrange the scones on a lined baking sheet. Bake for 15 minutes or until cooked through.

#7 Blueberry Avocado Chocolate Muffins

Serves: 9 muffins

Ingredients:

- 1 cup almond flour
- 1/2 cup almond milk (unsweetened)
- 1/3 cup coconut sugar
- 1/4 cup blueberries (fresh)
- 1/4 cup cacao powder + 1 tablespoon (raw)
- 2 large eggs (room temperature)
- 1/4 teaspoon salt
- 1 small avocado (ripe)
- 2 tablespoons coconut flour
- 2 tablespoons dark chocolate chips
- 2 teaspoons baking powder

Instructions:

- Pre-heat your oven to 375 degrees Fahrenheit. Line a muffin tin with muffin liners.
- In a blender, put in the eggs, sugar, avocado, salt, and 1 tablespoon of cacao powder. Blend them on high setting until the texture becomes like a smooth pudding. Transfer the mixture into a mixing bowl.

- In a mixing bowl, sift the coconut flour, baking powder, almond flour, and cocoa powder. Mix them well.
- Put in the almond milk into the avocado mixture. Get the flour mixture and fold it into the avocado mixture until combined. Do not overmix.
- Fold the chocolate chips and blueberries into the batter.
- Pour the batter evenly into the 9 cavities of the lined muffin tin.
- Bake for about 18 minutes or until cooked through. Let the muffins cool down before serving.

#8 Smoked Salmon in Scrambled Eggs

Serves: 2

Ingredients:

- 4 slices smoked salmon (chopped)
- 4 eggs
- 3 stems fresh chives (finely chopped)
- 2 tablespoons coconut milk
- Pinch of sea salt
- Cooking fat
- Pinch of black pepper (freshly ground)

Instructions:

- In a mixing bowl, put in the coconut milk, eggs, and chives. Whisk them together. Season with salt and pepper.
- In a skillet over medium heat, put in some cooking fat that is enough to cook the scrambled eggs.
- Pour the egg mixture onto the skillet. Stir to scramble the eggs.
- Stir in the salmon into the scrambled egg. Continue cooking for another 2 minutes. Serve.

#9 Tropical Smoothie Bowl

Serves: 2 bowls

Ingredients:

- 1 cup pineapple (frozen)
- 1 cup orange juice
- 1 cup mango (frozen)
- 1 spoonful of chia
- 1/2 banana
- 1/8 teaspoon turmeric

Toppings:

- Coconut flakes
- Kiwis (sliced)
- Strawberries (sliced)
- Almonds (chopped)

Instructions:

- In a blender, put in all the ingredients. Blend them until the texture becomes creamy and smooth. Adding a splash of orange juice at a time will help to smoothen up the mixture is it is too thick.
- Portion the smoothie equally between two bowls. Top each smoothie bowl with the listed toppings. Serve.

#10 Spinach and Potatoes with Smoked Salmon

Serves: 4

Ingredients:

- 4 eggs
- 2 russet potatoes (peeled and diced)
- 1/2 onion (sliced)
- 8 ounces smoked salmon (sliced)
- 2 cups baby spinach (fresh)
- 1/2 cup mushrooms (sliced)
- 1 garlic clove (minced)
- 2 tablespoons olive oil
- 2 tablespoons ghee
- 1/2 teaspoon onion powder
- 1/2 teaspoon garlic powder
- 1/4 teaspoon paprika
- Sea salt
- Black pepper

Instructions:

- Pre-heat your oven to 425 degrees Fahrenheit. Line a baking dish with parchment paper.
- Put the russet potatoes on the lined baking dish. Drizzle the potatoes with olive oil, paprika, garlic powder, and

onion powder. Season with salt and pepper.
- Bake the russet potatoes for 30 minutes. Turn the potatoes over halfway through the baking time.
- In a pot over high heat, put in some water. Bring the water to a boil.
- Put the eggs into the boiling water. Turn off the heat. Let the eggs cook in the hot water for 7 minutes.
- Take the eggs out from the pot. Let tap water run over the cooked eggs. Peel the eggs.
- In a saucepan over medium heat, put in the ghee and let it melt. Sautee the onion and garlic for a minute or two.
- Put in the mushrooms. Season with salt and pepper. Continue cooking for 5 minutes more.
- Put in the spinach. Cook for 2 minutes until they are wilted.
- Equally divide the russet potatoes into 4 portions. Top each portion with the spinach mixture, smoked salmon, and an egg. Serve.

#11 Bacon Avocado Burger

Serves: 1 burger

Ingredients:

- 2 bacon rashers
- 1 ripe avocado
- 1 red onion (sliced)
- 1 egg
- 1 lettuce leaf
- 1 tomato (sliced)
- 1 tablespoon Paleo mayonnaise
- Sesame seeds (for garnishing)
- Sea salt

Instructions:

- Put the bacon rashers on a frying pan. Turn on the stove to medium heat. Fry the bacon. Flip the bacon rashers using a fork when they are starting to curl. Continue cooking until they are crispy. Set aside the crispy bacon.
- Using the same frying pan, crack the egg on it. Cook the egg using the bacon fat. The egg white should have set but the egg yolk should still be runny. Set aside the cooked egg.

- Cut the avocado in half along its width. Take out the pit. Scoop the flesh from the skin using a spoon.
- Fill up the hole in the avocado with the mayonnaise.
- Layer on top of the avocado the lettuce, onion, tomato , bacon, and egg. Season with salt. Top the layer with the other half of the avocado.
- Garnish with sesame seeds. Serve.
-

#12 Bacon and Eggs in a Mushroom
Serves: 4

Ingredients:

- 4 pasture-raised eggs (large)
- 4 portobello mushroom caps
- 2 strips thick-cut and pasture-raised bacon (cooked and chopped)
- 1 medium tomato (chopped)
- 1 cup arugula
- Salt
- Pepper

Instructions:

- Pre-heat your oven to 350 degrees Fahrenheit. Prepare a baking tray. Line it with parchment paper.

- Take out the gills from the mushrooms using a spoon. Discard the gills.
- Arrange the mushrooms on the lined baking tray. Fill each mushroom cap with arugula and chopped tomatoes. Carefully crack an egg on top of each mushroom cap.
- Bake the mushrooms for 20 minutes in the middle rack.
- Top each mushroom with bacon, pepper, and salt. Serve.

#13 Tomato Mushroom & Spinach Fry Up

Serves: 2

Ingredients:

- 6 button mushrooms (sliced)
- 3 large handfuls of English spinach leaves (torn)
- Handful of cherry tomatoes (sliced in halves)
- 1/2 red onion (sliced)
- 1 garlic clove (finely diced)
- 2 tablespoons olive oil
- 1 teaspoon ghee
- 1/2 teaspoon lemon zest (grated)
- 1/2 teaspoon sea salt
- Pinch of nutmeg
- Pinch of black pepper (ground)
- Drizzle of lemon juice

Instructions:

- In a frying pan over medium heat, put in the ghee and olive oil. Sautee the onions and mushrooms until cooked through.
- Stir in the tomatoes, garlic, and lemon zest. Season with nutmeg, pepper, and salt. Continue cooking for 2 minutes

more. Smash the tomatoes using the spatula.
- Stir in the spinach leaves. Cook them until they are wilted. Drizzle with lemon juice. Serve.

#14 Almond Sweet Cherry Chia Pudding

Serves: 4 glasses

Ingredients:

- 2 cups whole sweet cherries (pitted)
- 3/4 cup chia seeds
- 1/2 cup hemp seeds
- 1/4 cup maple syrup
- 13.5 ounces can coconut milk
- 1 teaspoon vanilla extract
- 1 teaspoon almond extract
- 1/8 teaspoon sea salt

Topping:

- 4 cups cherries (halved and pitted)

Instructions:

- In a blender, put in the cherries, almond extract, coconut milk, vanilla extract,

maple syrup, and salt. Blend them until smooth.
- Put in the hemp seeds and chia seeds. Blend on low setting to combine.
- Pour the mixture equally among 4 glasses. Chill the pudding in the fridge for at least an hour.
- Top each pudding with cherries. Serve.

#15 Chocolate Milkshake
Serves: 1

Ingredients:

- 2 large organic bananas (frozen)
- 4 ice cubes
- 1 cup coconut milk
- 1 tablespoon cacao powder (raw)
- 2 tablespoons cashew butter
- 1/2 teaspoon vanilla extract

Instructions:

- In a food processor, put in the coconut milk and bananas. Pulse 2 – 3 times.
- Put in the cacao powder, cashew butter, and vanilla. Pulse again for 2 – 3 times.
- Put in the ice cubes. Blend until the mixture becomes smooth. You can add

more coconut milk or ice cubes to get a milkshake consistency that you like.
- Pour into a glass. Serve.

#16 Shakshuka
Serves: 6

Ingredients:

- 4 cups tomatoes (diced)
- 6 eggs (large)
- 1/2 onion (chopped)
- 1 red bell pepper (seeded and chopped)
- 1 clove garlic (minced)
- 2 tablespoons tomato paste
- 1 tablespoon cooking fat
- 1/2 tablespoon fresh parsley (finely chopped)
- 1 teaspoon paprika
- 1 teaspoon chilli powder
- Pinch of cayenne pepper
- Black pepper
- Sea salt

Instructions:

- In a skillet over medium heat, put in the cooking fat. Sautee the onions for 2

minutes. Put in the garlic. Continue sautéing until the onions are tender.
- Stir in the bell pepper. Continue cooking until the peppers are cooked.
- Stir in the tomatoes, tomato paste, paprika, chilli powder, and cayenne pepper. Season with salt and pepper.
- Reduce the heat. Let the mixture simmer for a few minutes.
- Crack the eggs on top of the simmering mixture. Space evenly the eggs. Cover the skillet. Let it simmer until the eggs are cooked through.
- Garnish with parsley. Serve.

#17 Amaranth Porridge with Pears
Serves: 2 bowls

Ingredients:

Porridge:

- 1/2 cup water
- 1/2 cup amaranth (uncooked, drained, and rinsed)
- 1/4 teaspoon salt
- 1 cup 2% milk

Pears:

- 1 pear (large and diced)
- 1 teaspoon maple syrup
- 1/2 teaspoon cinnamon (ground)
- 1/8 teaspoon nutmeg (ground)
- 1/4 teaspoon ginger (ground)
- 1/8 teaspoon clove (ground)

Topping:

- 2 tablespoons pecan pieces
- 1 cup 0% Greek yogurt (plain)
- 1 teaspoon maple syrup (pure)

Instructions:

- Preheat your oven to 400 degrees Fahrenheit. Line a baking sheet with parchment paper.
- In a pot over medium heat, put in the porridge ingredients. Bring to a boil. Lower the heat. Let the porridge simmer for 25 minutes. Set aside.
- Put the pecan pieces on the lined baking sheet. Coat them with maple syrup. Put the diced pears on the lined baking sheet beside the pecan pieces. Coat the pears with maple syrup. Roast them in the oven for 15 minutes.

- Stir in the pears into the porridge. Leave some pears for topping.
- Get two porridge bowls. Divide the yogurt between the two bowls. Scoop the porridge into each bowl. Top each bowl of porridge with pecans and the rest of the pears. Serve.

#18 Anti-Inflammatory Salad
Serves: 6

Ingredients:

Salad:

- 2 12-ounce bags of Trader Joe's Sweet Kale Salad Mix
- 16 ounces beets (cooked, peeled, and chopped)
- 1 1/2 cup blueberries (fresh)

Dressing:

- 1/3 cup extra virgin olive oil
- 1 clove garlic (grated)
- 2 tablespoons apple cider vinegar
- 1 teaspoon turmeric
- 1 tablespoon lemon juice
- 1 teaspoon fresh ginger (grated)

- 1/4 teaspoon black pepper (freshly ground)
- 1/2 teaspoon sea salt

Instructions:

- In a blender, put in the ingredients for the dressing. Blend until smooth.
- Divide the salad ingredients among 6 bowls. Drizzle with the dressing. Serve.

#19 Sweet Potato Breakfast Bowl
Serves: 1

Ingredients:

- 1 small banana (sliced)
- 1 small sweet potato (pre-baked)
- 1/4 cup raspberries
- 1 serving protein powder
- 1/4 cup blueberries

Toppings:

- Chia seeds
- Cacao nibs
- Favorite nuts
- Hemp hearts

Instructions:

- In a bowl, mash the flesh of the sweet potato. Put in the protein powder. Mix.
- Layer on top the bananas, blueberries, and raspberries.
- Put the toppings next. Serve.

#20 Overnight Oats with Almonds and Blueberries

Serves: 1

Ingredients:

Oats:

- 3/4 cup almond milk
- 3/4 cup old-fashioned oats
- 1 tablespoon maple syrup

Toppings:

- 1/3 cup yogurt
- 1/4 cup blueberries
- 3 tablespoons almonds (sliced)

Instructions:

- Put the oats in a mason jar (1-pint).

- In a mixing bowl, mix well the maple syrup and almond milk.
- Stir in the milk mixture into the oats. Seal the jar. Put in the fridge for at least 8 hours or overnight.
- Put the toppings. Serve.

#21 Apple Turkey Hash
Serves: 5

Ingredients:

Meat:

- 1 pound ground turkey
- 1/2 teaspoon thyme (dried)
- 1 tablespoon coconut oil
- Sea salt
- 1/2 teaspoon cinnamon

Hash:

- 2 cups frozen butternut squash (cubed)
- 2 cups spinach
- 1/2 cup carrots (shredded)
- 1 onion
- 1 large apple (peeled, cored, and chopped)
- 1 large zucchini
- 1 tablespoon coconut oil

- 1 teaspoon cinnamon
- 1/2 teaspoon garlic powder
- 3/4 teaspoon powdered ginger
- 1/2 teaspoon turmeric
- Sea salt
- 1/2 teaspoon thyme (dried)

Instructions:

- In a skillet over medium heat, put in the coconut oil. Stir in the ground turkey until cooked through. Season with thyme, cinnamon, and salt. Set aside.
- In the same skillet over medium heat, put in the coconut oil. Sautee the onions until softened.
- Stir in the carrots, zucchini, butternut squash, and apple. Cook them until they are softened.
- Stir in the spinach. Cook until wilted.
- Stir in the ground turkey and the rest of the seasonings. Serve.

#22 Chia Energy Bars with Chocolate

Serves: 14 bars

Ingredients:

- 1 1/2 cups pitted dates (packed)
- 1 cup walnut pieces (raw)
- 1/3 cup cacao powder (raw)
- 1/2 cup shredded coconut (unsweetened)
- 1/2 cup whole chia seeds
- 1/2 cup oats
- 1/2 cup dark chocolate (chopped)
- 1 teaspoon pure vanilla extract
- 1/4 teaspoon sea salt (unrefined)

Instructions:

- In a food processor, put in the dates. Process until it becomes a thick paste. Transfer it into a mixing bowl.
- Put in the walnuts. Mix thoroughly.
- Put in the remaining ingredients. Mix thoroughly until it becomes dough.
- Get a square baking pan. Line it with parchment paper. Transfer the dough on the lined pan. Spread the dough and press firmly into the pan.
- Put in the freezer for a few hours or overnight.

- Slice into 14 bars. Serve.

#23 Banana Chia Pudding

Serves: 3 glasses

Ingredients:

- 2 cups almond milk (unsweetened)
- 1/2 cup chia seeds
- 1 large banana (very ripe)
- 2 tablespoon maple syrup
- 1/2 teaspoon pure vanilla extract
- 1 tablespoon cacao powder

Mix-ins:

- 2 tablespoons cacao nibs
- 2 tablespoons chocolate chips
- 1 large banana (sliced)

Instructions:

- In a mixing bowl, put in the chia seeds and banana. Mash them well to combine.
- Put in the vanilla extract and milk. Whisk together until there are no more lumps.
- Prepare two containers with lid. Put half of the chia seeds mixture into one container. Cover.

- Stir in the cacao powder and maple syrup into the remaining half of the chia seeds mixture. Mix well. Put the mixture into the second container. Cover.
- Put both containers in the fridge for a few hours or overnight.
- Layer the chia seeds pudding equally among 3 glasses together with the mix-ins. Serve.

#24 Baked Rice Porridge with Maple and Fruit

Serves: 2 bowls

Ingredients:

- 1/2 cup brown rice
- 2 tablespoons pure maple syrup
- 1/2 teaspoon pure vanilla extract
- Sliced fruits (plums, berries, cherries, or pears)
- Pinch of cinnamon
- Pinch of salt

Instructions:

- Preheat your oven to 400 degrees Fahrenheit.

- In a pot over medium heat, put in a cup of water together with the brown rice. Bring to a boil.
- Stir in the cinnamon and vanilla extract. Cover. Lower the heat. Let the rice simmer until cooked. Stir the rice when needed.
- Get two oven-safe bowls. Divide the rice equally between the bowls. Top the rice with sliced fruits and maple syrup. Season with salt.
- Bake for 15 minutes. Serve.

#25 Baked Eggs with Herbs
Serves: 1

Ingredients:

- 2 eggs
- 1 tablespoon milk
- 1 teaspoon butter (melted)
- Sprinkle of dried thyme, garlic powder, dried parsley, dried oregano, and dried dill

Instructions:

- Pre-heat your oven to Broil in low setting.

- In a small baking dish, put in the milk and butter. Mix well. Coat the baking dish with the butter-milk mixture.
- Crack the eggs into the baking dish. Sprinkle with the herbs and garlic.
- Bake for a few minutes until the eggs are cooked.

#26 Cinnamon Granola with Fruits

Serves: 3 1/2 cups

Ingredients:

- 2 cups old-fashioned rolled oats
- 1/4 cup walnuts (chopped)
- 1/4 cup shredded coconut (unsweetened)
- 1/4 cup honey
- 1/4 cup dried apricots (chopped)
- 1/4 cup raisins
- 1/4 cup dried cranberries
- 4 tablespoons unsalted butter (melted)
- 2 tablespoons pumpkin seeds
- 1/2 teaspoon ground cinnamon
- 1/4 teaspoon ground nutmeg
- 1/4 teaspoon ground cloves

Instructions:

- Pre-heat your oven to 300 degrees Fahrenheit. Line a baking tray with parchment paper.
- In a mixing bowl, put in the coconuts, pumpkin seeds, walnuts, spices, and oats. Set aside.
- In another bowl, put in the butter and honey. Mix well. Pour the mixture into the oat mixture. Mix well.
- Transfer the oat mixture on the lined baking tray. Spread evenly. Bake for 25 minutes.
- Let it cool down. Crumble the granola. Mix the crumbled granola with the dried fruits. Store in an airtight container.

#27 Banana Bread Pecan Overnight Oats

Serves: 2 bowls

Ingredients:

- 1 1/2 cups milk
- 1 cup old-fashioned rolled oats
- 1/4 cup Greek yogurt (plain)
- 2 bananas (very ripe, mashed)
- 2 tablespoons honey

- 2 tablespoons coconut flakes (unsweetened, toasted)
- 1 tablespoon chia seeds
- 1/4 teaspoon sea salt (flaked)
- 2 teaspoons vanilla extract

Topping:

- Roasted pecans
- Banana slices
- Honey
- Fig halves
- Pomegranate seeds

Instructions:

- In a mixing bowl, put in the oats, bananas, milk, coconut flakes, yogurt, chia seeds, honey, sea salt, and vanilla extract. Mix well to combine.
- Equally divide the oat mixture between two bowls. Cover. Put in the fridge for at least 6 hours or overnight.
- Stir the mixture. Top each bowl of oats with the toppings. Serve.

#28 Yogurt Parfait with Chia Seeds and Raspberries

Serves: 2 glasses

Ingredients:

- 1/2 cup raspberries (fresh)
- 16 ounces yogurt (plain, divided into 4 portions)
- 2 tablespoons chia seeds
- Pinch of cinnamon
- 1 teaspoon maple syrup

Topping:

- Blackberries (sliced)
- Strawberries (sliced)
- Nectarines (sliced)

Instructions:

- In a mixing bowl, put in the raspberries. Mash them until they look like a jam.
- Put in the honey, chia seeds, and cinnamon. Mash them all together until well combined. Portion into 2 equal parts.
- Get two glasses. Layer each glass with a portion of yogurt at the bottom. The next layer is the raspberry mixture. The last layer is the remaining portions of yogurt.
- Put the toppings. Serve.

#29 Winter Morning Breakfast Bowl

Serves: 2 bowls

Ingredients:

- 2 1/2 cups coconut water
- 1 cup of quinoa
- 2 whole cloves
- 1 cinnamon stick
- 1 star anise pod

Fresh Fruits:

- Apples
- Blackberries
- Cranberries
- Pears
- Persimmons

Instructions:

- In a saucepan over medium heat, put in the quinoa, coconut water, and spices. Bring them to a boil.
- Cover the pan. Lower the heat. Let it simmer for 25 minutes.
- Equally divide the quinoa between two bowls. Remove the whole spices.
- Top each bowl with fresh fruits. Serve.

#30 Avocado Toast with Egg
Serves: 1

Ingredients:

- 1 1/2 teaspoon ghee
- 1 slice gluten-free bread (toasted)
- 1 egg (scrambled)
- 1/2 avocado (sliced)
- Red pepper flakes
- Handful of spinach leaves

Instructions:

- Top the toasted bread with ghee.
- Arrange the avocado slices on the bread.
- Top with spinach leaves.
- Put the scrambled egg on top.
- Sprinkle with red pepper flakes. Serve.

Chapter 7: Anti-Inflammatory Lunch Recipes

#1 Avocado Chickpea Salad Sandwich

Serves: 2 sandwiches

Ingredients:

- 1 large avocado (ripe)
- 1 15-ounce-can chickpeas (rinsed and drained)
- 2 teaspoons lemon juice (freshly squeezed)
- 4 slices whole grain bread
- 1/4 cup cranberries (dried)
- Salt
- Freshly ground pepper

Toppings:

- Red onion
- Arugula
- Spinach

Instructions:

- In a mixing bowl, put in the chickpeas. Smash them using a fork. Put in the avocado. Continue to smash until the texture is smooth with some chunky pieces.
- Put in the cranberries and lemon juice. Season with pepper and salt. Mix well.
- Toast the bread slices. Portion the chickpea mixture into two equal parts. Spread each portion over a slice of bread. Top with any topping of your choice. Put a slice of bread on top to complete the sandwich. Serve.

#2 Buddha Bowl with Avocado, Kale, Wild Rice, and Orange

Serves: 2 bowls

Ingredients:

Rice:

- 3 cups vegetable broth
- 1 cup wild rice
- 1 garlic clove (minced)
- 2 tablespoons rice vinegar
- 2 tablespoons extra-virgin olive oil

- 1 tablespoon fresh mint (chopped)
- Freshly ground black pepper
- Salt

Toppings:

- 1/4 cup pomegranate seeds
- 1/4 cup pumpkin seeds
- 1 bunch kale (roughly chopped)
- 2 eggs (hard-boiled)
- 1 orange (segmented)
- 1/2 avocado (sliced)
- 1 tablespoon rice vinegar
- 2 tablespoons olive oil
- Freshly ground black pepper
- Salt

Instructions:

Rice:

- In a pot over medium heat, put in the broth, rice, and garlic. Stir to combine. Bring it to a boil. Lower the heat. Simmer the rice for 15 minutes or until tender and no more liquid left.
- Set aside the rice for 10 minutes to cool down. Put in the mint, vinegar, olive oil, pepper, and salt. Toss to combine well with the rice.

Toppings:

- In a mixing bowl, put in the kale, vinegar, and olive oil. Toss to mix well.
- Portion the rice equally between two bowls. Top each rice bowl with kale mixture.
- Divide the rest of the toppings equally between the two bowls. Season with pepper and salt. Serve.

#3 Spiced Lentil Soup
Serves: 7 cups

Ingredients:

- 3 1/2 cups vegetable broth (low-sodium)
- 3/4 cup red lentils (uncooked, rinsed, and drained)
- 1 1/2 tablespoons extra-virgin olive oil
- 2 garlic cloves (minced)
- 1 large onion (diced)
- 1 14-ounce-can coconut milk (full-fat)
- 1 14-ounce-can diced tomatoes (with juice)
- 1 5-ounce-package baby spinach
- 2 teaspoons turmeric (ground)
- 2 teaspoons fresh lime juice
- 1 1/2 teaspoons cumin (ground)

- 1/2 teaspoon fine sea salt
- 1/2 teaspoon cinnamon
- 1/4 teaspoon cardamom (ground)
- Cayenne pepper
- Freshly ground black pepper

Instructions:

- In a pot over medium heat, put in the oil. Sautee the garlic, onion, and salt until the onion is soft.
- Put in the cardamom, cinnamon, cumin, and turmeric. Stir to combine. Cook for another minute.
- Put in the tomatoes, coconut milk, broth, red lentils, cayenne, pepper, and salt. Stir to combine very well. Bring the mixture to a boil.
- Lower the heat. Let the mixture simmer for 20 minutes. The le ntils should be tender and fluffy.
- Remove the pot from the heat. Put in the spinach. Stir to combine. Season with lime juice, salt, and pepper. Serve.

#4 Tuna Mediterranean Salad

Serves: 6

Ingredients:

- 2 cans Albacore Tuna (drained)
- 1 14.5-ounce-can chickpeas (drained and rinsed)
- 1 cup red peppers (roasted and chopped)
- 1/3 cup parsley (finely chopped)
- 1/2 cup pepperocini (diced)
- 1/4 cup feta cheese
- 1/2 red onion (diced)
- 1 cucumber (chopped)
- 2 teaspoons capers
- Olives
- Sundried tomatoes (chopped)
- Pinch of black pepper
- Pinch of fine sea salt

Dressing:

- 2 tablespoons red wine vinegar
- 2 tablespoons olive oil
- 1 teaspoon lemon juice
- 1 teaspoon dried oregano
- 1 teaspoon dried parsley
- Pinch black pepper
- Pinch fine salt

Instructions:

- In a mixing bowl, put all the salad ingredients.
- In another bowl, put in all the dressing ingredients. Whisk well.
- Pour the dressing on the salad. Toss to combine everything.
- Serve together with 1/2 avocado.

#5 Red Lentil Pasta with Tomato

Serves: 6 bowls

Ingredients:

- 1/2 cup sun-dried tomatoes (oil packed, drained and chopped)
- 1/4 cup extra virgin olive oil
- 6 cloves garlic (minced)
- 1 sweet onion (chopped)
- 2 large handfuls kale
- 1 can (28 ounces) fire roasted tomatoes
- 1 box (8 ounces) red lentil pasta
- 1 tablespoon oregano (dried)
- 1 tablespoon basil (dried)
- 1 tablespoon apple cider vinegar
- 2 teaspoons turmeric (ground)
- Pepper

- Kosher salt
- Toasted pine nuts (for topping)

Instructions:

- In a pot over medium heat, put in the oil. Sautee the onion for 5 minutes until soft.
- Stir in the garlic, oregano, basil, turmeric, pepper, and salt. Cook for another minute.
- Stir in the roasted tomatoes (juice included). Crush the tomatoes while stirring.
- Put in the sun-dried tomatoes and vinegar. Let the mixture simmer for 15 minutes.
- Stir in the kale. Continue cooking for 5 minutes more.
- Cook the red lentil pasta according to package directions.
- Equally portion the pasta among 6 bowls. Top each bowl with the tomato sauce and pine nuts. Serve.

#6 Chicken and Greek Salad Wrap

Serves: 2 wraps

Ingredients:

Chicken:

- 2 chicken breasts (bone-in)
- 1 tablespoon olive oil (divided)
- 1/2 teaspoon dried oregano
- 1/2 teaspoon garlic powder
- 1/2 teaspoon lemon pepper

Salad:

- 4 cups romaine (chopped)
- 1/3 cup feta cheese
- 1/3 cup cherry tomatoes (sliced)
- 1/2 cup cucumber slices (chopped)
- 1/4 cup red onion
- 4 tablespoons hummus
- 2 tablespoons kalamata olives
- 1/2 teaspoon dried oregano
- 2 gluten free wraps
- 1 fresh lemon wedge (juiced)
- olive oil
- red wine vinegar

Instructions:

Chicken:

- Pre-heat your oven to 375 degrees Fahrenheit. Line a baking tray with foil. Drizzle with half of the olive oil.
- Put the chicken on the lined baking tray. Season with lemon pepper, oregano, garlic powder, pepper, and salt. Drizzle with the other half of the olive oil.
- Bake for 40 minutes until cooked. Let the chicken cool completely. Slice to bite sizes.

Salad:

- In a mixing bowl, put in the romaine, tomatoes, cucumbers, onion, olives, cheese, and oregano.
- Dress the salad with two turns of the vinegar around the bowl, one turn of the olive oil, and lemon juice. Toss to combine.

Wrap:

- Spread 2 tablespoons of hummus on each wrap. Layer the chicken slices and salad on top. Wrap. Serve.

#7 Butternut Squash Carrot Soup

Serves: 4 bowls

Ingredients:

- 1 1/2 pounds butternut squash (peeled and chopped)
- 1 pound carrots (chopped)
- 4 cups vegetable stock
- 1/2 cup shallots (sliced)
- 1 can coconut milk (full-fat)
- 2 tablespoons avocado oil
- 1 tablespoon fresh ginger (grated)
- Freshly ground black pepper
- 1 teaspoon salt

Garnishing:

- Coconut milk
- Roasted chickpeas
- Cilantro

Instructions:

- Pre-heat your oven to 400 degrees Fahrenheit. Line a baking sheet with parchment paper.
- Put on the lined baking sheet the butternut squash, carrots, and shallots.
- Drizzle with oil. Season with salt. Lightly toss the vegetables to coat.

- Roast them for 30 minutes. Let them cool down for a few minutes.
- In a blender, put in the roasted vegetables, coconut milk, vegetable stock, ginger, pepper, and salt. Blend until creamy in texture.
- Divide the soup among 4 bowls. Garnish each bowl with coconut milk, chickpeas, and cilantro.

#8 Cauliflower and Chickpea Coconut Curry

Serves: 4

Ingredients:

- 1 can (28 ounces) cooked chickpeas
- 1 can (14 ounces) coconut milk
- 1 1/2 cups frozen peas
- 1/4 cup fresh cilantro (chopped)
- 4 scallions (thinly sliced)
- 1 red bell pepper (thinly sliced)
- 1 red onion (thinly sliced)
- 1 lime (halved)
- 1 small head cauliflower (bite-size florets)
- 3 garlic cloves (minced)
- 3 tablespoons red curry paste
- 1 tablespoon fresh ginger (minced)

- 1 tablespoon extra-virgin olive oil
- 1 teaspoon ground coriander
- 2 teaspoons chilli powder
- Freshly ground black pepper
- Salt

Instructions:

- In a pot over medium heat, put in the oil. Sautee the onion and bell pepper for 5 minutes. Put in the garlic and ginger. Sautee for another minute.
- Put in the cauliflower, coriander, chilli powder, and curry paste. Cook for a minute.
- Put in the coconut milk. Stir. Simmer the mixture over low heat until the cauliflower is tender.
- Juice the lime into the curry. Stir. Put in the peas and chickpeas. Season with pepper and salt. Let it simmer for a few minutes.
- Garnish each serving with a tablespoon of scallions and cilantro. Serve.

#9 Kale Quinoa Shrimp Bowl

Serves: 4 bowls

Ingredients:

Kale:

- 1 bunch lacinato kale (roughly torn)
- 2 tablespoons extra-virgin olive oil
- Freshly ground black pepper
- Salt

Quinoa:

- 2 cups chicken broth
- 1 1/4 cups quinoa
- 2 teaspoons extra-virgin olive oil
- Freshly ground pepper
- Salt

Shrimp and Toppings:

- 1 pound shrimp (peeled and deveined)
- 2 watermelon radishes (thinly sliced)
- 2 avocados (sliced)
- 2 tablespoons hot sauce
- 1 tablespoon extra-virgin olive oil
- 3/4 teaspoon ground coriander
- 1 teaspoon ground cumin
- Freshly ground black pepper
- Salt

Instructions:

Kale:

- Pre-heat your oven to 400 degrees Fahrenheit. Line a baking tray with parchment paper.
- In a mixing bowl, put in the kale and olive oil. Season with pepper and salt. Toss to combine.
- Put the kale in a single layer on the lined baking tray. Roast for 17 minutes until very crispy.

Quinoa:

- In a pot over medium heat, put in the olive oil. Stir in the quinoa. Toast it for a minute.
- Put in the broth. Let the quinoa simmer until tender. Season with pepper and salt.

Shrimp:

- In a skillet over medium heat, put in the olive oil.
- In a mixing bowl, put in the shrimp, cumin, hot sauce, coriander, pepper, and salt. Toss to combine.
- Sautee the shrimp mixture on the heated skillet for 5 minutes until cooked.

Bowls:

- Divide the cooked quinoa among 4 bowls. Top each bowl with crispy kale, shrimp, avocado slices, and watermelon radishes. Serve.

#10 Turkey Taco Bowls

Serves: 4 bowls

Ingredients:

Rice:

- 1/8 teaspoon salt
- 3/4 cup brown rice (uncooked)
- 1 lime (zested)

Turkey:

- 3/4 pound ground turkey (lean)
- 2/3 cup water
- 2 tablespoons taco seasoning

Salsa:

- 1 pint cherry tomatoes (halved)
- 1/4 cup red onion (finely chopped)
- 1 jalapeno (finely chopped)
- 1/8 teaspoon salt

- 1/2 lime (juiced)

Topping:

- 1/2 cup mozzarella (shredded)
- 1 can (12 ounces) corn kernels (drained)

Instructions:

- Cook the brown rice following the instructions from the package. Just put in salt and lime zest to the cooking water. Set aside the cooked rice to cool down a bit.
- In a pan over medium heat, put in the turkey. Cook the turkey for 10 minutes until the color is no longer pink.
- Put in the taco seasoning and water. Stir to combine. Let the mixture simmer for 2 minutes to thicken the sauce. Set aside the turkey to cool down a bit.
- In a mixing bowl, put in all the ingredients for the salsa. Toss to combine everything.
- Portion the rice among 4 bowls. Top each rice bowl with the turkey and salsa. Put the mozzarella and corn kernels as toppings.Serve.

#11 Veggies and Egg Bowl

Serves: 4 bowls

Ingredients:

- 1 pound sweet potatoes (diced)
- 1 pound Brussels sprouts (cut in half)
- 4 eggs (poached)
- 2 cups arugula
- 3 tablespoons apple cider vinegar
- 2 tablespoons harissa
- 1 1/2 tablespoons olive oil

Instructions:

- Preheat your oven to 400 degrees Fahrenheit. Line a baking tray with parchment paper.
- Evenly spread the sweet potatoes and Brussels sprouts on the lined baking tray. Drizzle with olive oil. Season with pepper and salt.
- Roast for 20 minutes until tender.
- In a mixing bowl, mix together the apple cider vinegar, olive oil, and harissa.
- Portion the roasted vegetables among 4 bowls. Top each bowl with arugula, an egg, and the harissa dressing. Serve.

#12 Bulgur Kale Pesto Salad

Serves: 4

Ingredients:

- 1/2 pound green beans (trimmed and bite-size slices)
- 1 1/2 cups bulgur
- 1/2 cup packed basil leaves
- 1 cup lacinato kale (stemmed and thinly sliced)
- 1/4 cup plus 3 tablespoons almonds (sliced and toasted)
- 1/4 cup lemon juice
- 1/4 cup extra-virgin olive oil
- 1 pint grape tomatoes (halved)
- 1/4 packed flat-leaf parsley
- 1 garlic clove
- 3 tablespoons almonds (sliced)
- 1 teaspoon kosher salt (divided)
- 1/4 teaspoon ground black pepper
- 1/2 teaspoon kosher salt

Instructions:

Salad:

- In a bowl, put in 3 cups water, 1/2 teaspoon salt, and bulgur. Let the bulgur soak overnight. Drain the excess liquid.

Pesto:

- In a food processor, put in the garlic. Pulse until chopped. Put in the basil, kale, 1/4 cup almonds, and parsley. Pulse until chopped finely. Put in the lemon juice, pepper, and 1/2 teaspoon salt. Puree the mixture until smooth.
- Pour the pesto into the bulgur. Put in green beans, tomatoes, and the remaining toasted almonds. Toss. Top with the almond slices. Serve.

#13 Swiss Chard and Red Lentil Curried Soup

Serves: 6

Ingredients:

- 1 pound Swiss chard (tough stalks removed and chopped coarsely)
- 2 cups dried red lentils
- 5 cups vegetable broth
- 1 can (15 ounces) chickpeas (rinsed and drained)
- 6 tablespoons thick Greek yogurt (thinned with 2 tablespoons water)
- 5 teaspoons curry powder
- 2 tablespoons olive oil

- 1 large onion (thinly sliced)
- 1 lime (sliced into 6 wedges)
- 1 red jalapeño chili (stemmed and thinly sliced)
- 1/4 teaspoon ground cayenne pepper
- 1 teaspoon salt

Instructions:

- In a saucepan over medium heat, put in the oil. Sautee the onion for 10 minutes until lightly golden.
- Stir in the cayenne and curry.
- Put in the chard and 4 cups broth. Let it boil with constant stirring until the chard is wilted.
- Stir in the chickpeas and lentils. Lower the heat. Let it simmer for 18 minutes until lentils are soft.
- Turn off heat. In a food processor, pour in about half of the soup. Puree it. Pour the puree back to the pot. Put in the salt and remaining broth. Stir. Warm the soup for a couple of minutes over low heat.
- Pour into 6 bowls. Garnish with yogurt, lime wedge, and jalapeño. Serve.

#14 Turkish Scrambled Eggs

Serves: 4

Ingredients:

- 6 eggs (beaten)
- 4 ripe tomatoes (diced)
- 4 whole grain pitas (serving)
- 3 scallions (finely chopped)
- 2 tablespoons olive oil
- 2 tablespoons fresh parsley (chopped)
- 2 large red bell peppers (seeded and finely chopped)
- 4 ounces Feta cheese (crumbled)
- 1 teaspoon red pepper flakes (crushed)
- 1/2 teaspoon kosher salt
- 1/4 teaspoon ground black pepper
- Green olives (garnish)

Instructions:

- In a skillet over medium heat, put in the oil. Sautee the scallions for two minutes until soft. Put in the peppers. Sautee for 5 minutes. Put in the pepper flakes and tomatoes. Sautee for 5 minutes more.
- Put in the cheese and eggs. Scramble with constant stirring. Cook until the eggs are done. Season with pepper and salt. Turn

off the heat. Stir in the parsley. Garnish with olives. Serve with pitas on the side.

#15 Orange Cardamom Quinoa with Carrots

Serves: 4

Ingredients:

- 1 pound carrots (peeled and sliced)
- 2 1/2 cups vegetable broth
- 1 cup quinoa (rinsed)
- 1/3 cup golden raisins
- 2 oranges (zested and segmented)
- 1-inch fresh ginger (peeled and minced)
- 1/2 teaspoon freshly ground black pepper
- 1 teaspoon ground cardamom
- 1/2 teaspoon salt

Instructions:

- In a slow cooker, put in the orange zest, black pepper, salt, cardamom, ginger, raisins, carrots, broth, and quinoa. Mix well. Cook for 3 1/2 hours on low setting.
- Divide the quinoa among 4 bowls. Top each bowl with some orange segments. Serve.

#16 Tomato Stew with Chickpea and Kale

Serves: 4

Ingredients:

- 1 pound tomatoes (cored and chopped)
- 3/4 pound kale (stemmed and leaves coarsely chopped)
- 1 cup vegetable stock
- 2 cans (15-ounce) chickpeas (drained and rinsed)
- 1 medium onion (sliced into eighths)
- 6 garlic cloves (thinly sliced)
- 4 large eggs
- 4 tablespoons olive oil (divided)
- 1 1/4 teaspoon kosher salt (divided)
- 1/4 teaspoon red pepper flakes (crushed)

Instructions:

- In a saucepan over medium heat, put in half of the oil. Put in the onion and half of the salt. Sautee the onions for 7 minutes. Stir in the pepper flakes and garlic. Sautee for 2 more minutes.
- Put in the kale. Cook until wilted. Put in the stock, chickpeas, and tomatoes. Cook for 10 minutes. Season with salt.

- In a skillet over medium heat, put in the remaining half of the oil. Crack an egg and cook until the white is set and the bottom is lightly crisp. Do the same with the rest of the eggs.
- Divide the stew among 4 bowls. Top with an egg. Season with salt. Serve.

#17 Quinoa Turmeric Power Bowl
Serves: 4 bowls

Ingredients:

- 7 small yellow potatoes (slice into strips)
- 2 kale leaves (rinsed)
- 1 avocado (sliced)
- 1/4 cup quinoa
- 1 can (15 ounces) chickpeas (drained and rinsed)
- 1 tablespoon coconut oil
- 1/2 tablespoon olive oil
- 1 teaspoon paprika
- 2 teaspoons turmeric(divided)
- Pepper
- Salt

Instructions:

- Preheat your oven to 350 degrees Fahrenheit.
- Lay flat the potato strips on the half part of a baking sheet. Drizzle with coconut oil. Season with a teaspoon of turmeric, pepper, and salt.
- Roast for 5 minutes.
- In a mixing bowl, put in the chickpeas and paprika. Toss to coat well. Spread the chickpeas on the other half of the baking sheet beside the potatoes.
- Roast for 25 minutes.
- In a pot over medium heat, put in half cup of water and quinoa. Cook the quinoa until tender. Season with a teaspoon of turmeric, pepper, and salt. Stir well. Set aside to cool.
- Massage the kale with olive oil. Divide the leaves among 4 bowls. Layer each bowl with avocado slices, quinoa, and roasted vegetables. Serve.

#18 Anti-Inflammatory Beef Meatballs

Serves: 4

Ingredients:

- 2 pounds ground beef
- 1/4 cup chopped cilantro (tightly packed)
- Zest of 1 lime
- 5 garlic cloves (pressed)
- 1/2 teaspoon sea salt
- 1/2 teaspoon ground ginger

Instructions:

- Preheat your oven to 350 degrees Fahrenheit. Line a baking tray with parchment paper.
- In a mixing bowl, put in all the ingredients. Mix well. Shape the mixture into 12 meatballs. Arrange the meatballs on the lined baking tray.
- Bake for 25 minutes until cooked. Serve the meatballs with cilantro, parsley, and avocado slices.

#19 Roasted Salmon Garlic and Broccoli

Serves: 4

Ingredients:

- 1 1/2 pounds salmon fillets (quartered and patted dry
- 1 lemon (sliced)
- 1 large broccoli head (sliced into florets)
- 2 cloves fresh garlic (minced)
- 2 1/2 tablespoons coconut oil (melted and divided)
- Black pepper
- 3/4 teaspoon sea salt (divided)

Instructions:

- Preheat your oven to 450 degrees Fahrenheit. Line a baking tray with parchment paper.
- Arrange the salmon on the lined baking tray. There should be some space in between each piece.
- Drizzle the salmon with a tablespoon of olive oil. Spread the garlic closely to the salmon pieces. Season with pepper and half of the salt. Put a slice of lemon on top of each salmon piece. Set aside.

- In a mixing bowl, put in the broccoli florets, the other half of the salt, pepper, and 1 1/2 tablespoons of oil. Toss. Arrange the florets in between each salmon piece.
- Bake for 15 minutes. Garnish with parsley and lemon slices. Serve.

#20 Salmon with Veggies Sheet Pan

Serves: 4

Ingredients:

- 16 ounces Brussels sprouts (halved)
- 16 ounces bag baby potatoes
- 4 6-ounce salmon fillets (skin on)
- 1/2 red onion (cubed)
- 1 cup cherry tomatoes
- 1 bunch asparagus (trimmed and halved)
- 1 garlic clove (minced)
- 3 tablespoons balsamic vinegar
- 2 tablespoons honey
- 2 tablespoons olive oil
- 1 tablespoon dijon mustard
- 1/2 teaspoon sea salt
- 1 teaspoon fresh thyme

Instructions:

- Preheat your oven to 450 degrees Fahrenheit. Line a baking sheet with parchment paper.
- In a bowl, put in the vinegar, honey, garlic, Dijon mustard, salt, and thyme. Mix well.
- In another bowl, put in the asparagus, Brussels sprouts, red onion, potatoes, olive oil, tomatoes, and 3 tablespoons of balsamic honey mixture. Mix well.
- Spread the vegetables evenly on the lined baking sheet.
- Bake for 10 minutes. Take out from the oven.
- Arrange the salmon fillets on the top of the vegetables. The skin side is down. Brush each fillet with the rest of the balsamic honey mixture.
- Put back the baking sheet in the oven. Bake for 10 minutes.
- Switch the oven setting to broiler high for 4 minutes. This will brown the fillet tops. Serve.

#21 Roasted Sweet Potatoes with Avocado Dip

Serves: 4

Ingredients:

- 2 large sweet potatoes (washed and cubed)
- 1 avocado (halved and pitted)
- 1 lime (juice)
- 1 large clove garlic (peeled and chopped)
- 4 tablespoons water
- 1/2 teaspoon sea salt (divided)
- 2 tablespoons olive oil
- 1 teaspoon olive oil

Instructions:

- Preheat your oven to 400 degrees Fahrenheit. Line a baking pan with parchment paper.
- Spread evenly the cubed potatoes on the lined baking pan. Drizzle with 2 tablespoons of olive oil.
- Flip each potato piece to make sure that the oil coats each piece.
- Season with half of the salt. Bake for 45 minutes until light brown in color.

- In a blender, put in the avocado, lime juice, garlic, and the other half of the salt. Blend until creamy.
- Gradually add in the water and olive oil. Continue to blend until mixed well.
- Serve the baked potatoes with the dip.

#22 Lentil Soup with Lemons
Serves: 8

Ingredients:

- 2 cups green lentils (washed and picked over for stones)
- 1 1/2 cups celery (diced)
- 1 1/2 cups carrots (diced)
- 2 1/2 boxes (32 ounces) vegetable broth
- 1 tablespoon extra virgin olive oil
- 3 cloves garlic (minced)
- 3 small lemons (juiced)
- 1 yellow onion (diced)
- 2 teaspoons dried turmeric
- 4 teaspoons fresh ginger (grated)
- 1 teaspoon salt
- Zest of 1/2 lemon

Instructions:

- In a Dutch oven over medium heat, put in the oil. Sautee the onion, celery, carrots, and salt for 5 minutes. Stir in the ginger and garlic. Cook for a minute more. Stir in the broth, lentils, and turmeric.
- Lower the heat. Let the soup simmer for 45 minutes, partially covered. Put in the lemon juice and zest. Stir. Simmer the soup for 30 minutes more. Serve.

#23 Chicken with Lemon and Asparagus
Serves: 4

Ingredients:

- 1 pound chicken breasts (boneless and skinless)
- 2 cups asparagus (chopped)
- 1/4 cup flour
- 4 tablespoons butter (divided)
- 2 lemons (sliced)
- 1 teaspoon lemon pepper seasoning
- 1/2 teaspoon pepper
- 1/2 teaspoon salt

Instructions:

Chicken:

- Cut each chicken breast in half resulting to 3/4 inch thick slices.
- In a shallow dish, put in the flour, pepper, and salt. Mix well. Coat each chicken slice with the flour mixture.
- In a skillet over medium heat, melt the first half of the butter. Put the chicken slices in. Cook for 5 minutes on each side until golden brown. Sprinkle each side of the chicken with lemon pepper while cooking. Set aside.

Lemons and Asparagus:

- In the same skillet over medium heat, melt the remaining butter. Put in the asparagus. Sautee until tender crisp. Take out from the pan.
- Arrange the lemon slices flat on the skillet over medium heat. Cook each side for a couple of minutes without stirring to caramelize. Take out from the pan.

Assembly:

- Layer the cooked ingredients on a platter – asparagus, chicken, and lemon. Serve.

#24 Shrimp Fajitas

Serves: 4

Ingredients:

- 1 1/2 pounds shrimp (peeled and deveined)
- 1 red bell pepper (sliced thinly)
- 1 yellow bell pepper (sliced thinly)
- 1 small red onion (sliced thinly)
- 1 orange bell pepper (sliced thinly)
- 1 1/2 tablespoons extra virgin olive oil
- 2 teaspoons chili powder
- 1 teaspoon kosher salt
- 1/2 teaspoon onion powder
- 1/2 teaspoon garlic powder
- 1/2 teaspoon smoked paprika
- 1/2 teaspoon ground cumin
- Freshly ground pepper
- Lime
- Tortillas (warmed)
- Fresh cilantro (for garnish)

Instructions:

- Preheat your oven to 450 degrees Fahrenheit. Grease a baking sheet with cooking spray.

- In a mixing bowl, put in shrimp, bell peppers, onion, olive oil, spices, pepper, and salt. Toss well.
- Spread them evenly on the greased baking sheet.
- Bake for 8 minutes. Switch the oven setting to Broil. Cook the fajita for another 2 minutes.
- Squeeze the lime juice over the fajita. Garnish with cilantro. Serve together with warm tortillas.

#25 Garlic Tomato Basil Chicken
Serves: 4

Ingredients:

- 1 pound chicken breasts (boneless and skinless)
- 4 medium zucchini (spiralized)
- 1 cup fresh basil (loosely packed and cut into ribbons)
- 14.5-ounce can chopped tomatoes
- 3 garlic cloves (minced)
- 1/2 yellow onion (diced)
- 2 tablespoons olive oil (divided)
- 1/4 teaspoon red pepper flakes (crushed)
- Salt

- Pepper

Instructions:

- Wrap each chicken breast with plastic wrap. Pound them to an even 1 inch thick all around. Unwrap each chicken breast. Season with pepper and salt.
- In a skillet over medium heat, put in a tablespoon of olive oil. Put the chicken breasts. Pan fry them until browned and cooked through. Set aside.
- In the same skillet over medium heat, put in the remaining olive oil. Sautee the onion for 5 minutes. Put in the garlic. Sautee for a minute more.
- Stir in the basil and tomatoes. Season with red pepper flakes, pepper, and salt. Let it simmer for 10 minutes with occasional stirring.
- Stir in the zoodles and chicken breasts. Simmer for a few minutes. Serve.

#26 Mediterranean One Pan Cod

Serves: 4

Ingredients:

- 2 cups kale (shredded)
- 2 cups fennel (sliced)
- 1 cup fresh tomatoes (diced)
- 1 cup oil cured black olives
- 1/2 cup water
- 1 pound cod (quartered)
- 1 small onion (sliced)
- 1 can (14.5 ounces) diced tomato
- 3 large cloves garlic (chopped)
- 2 tablespoons olive oil
- 1 teaspoon orange zest
- 1/2 teaspoon dried oregano
- 1/4 teaspoon fennel seeds
- 1/4 teaspoon black pepper
- 1/8 teaspoon salt
- Pinch of red pepper (crushed)

Garnish:

- Fennel fronds
- Fresh oregano
- Olive oil
- Orange zest

Instructions:

- In a skillet over medium heat, put in the olive oil. Cook the onion, garlic, and fennel for 8 minutes. Season with pepper and salt.
- Stir in the canned tomatoes, fresh tomatoes, water, and kale. Cook for 12 minutes more. Stir in the oregano, red pepper, and olives.
- Season the cod with pepper, salt, fennel seeds, and zest. Arrange the fish on top of the tomato mixture. Cover the skillet. Simmer for 10 minutes.
- Garnish. Serve.

#27 Asian Garlic Noodles
Serves: 4

Ingredients:

Noodles:

- 1 large spaghetti squash
- 1 small red bell pepper (minced)
- 1/2 large carrot (julienne cut)
- 1/2 medium zucchini (julienne cut)
- 1/4 cup roasted cashews (chopped)
- 1/2 cup fresh cilantro (diced)

Sauce:

- 6 large medjool dates (pitted)
- 6 garlic cloves
- 1/4 cup coconut milk (full fat)
- 2/3 cup coconut aminos
- 2 tablespoons red curry paste
- 2 tablespoons fresh ginger (grated)
- 2 tablespoons fish sauce

Instructions:

- Pre-heat your oven to 450 degrees Fahrenheit.
- Slice the spaghetti squash in half lengthwise. Scrape off the seeds.
- Put the spaghetti squash on a baking tray facing up. Brush the exposed surface with olive oil.
- Bake for 25 minutes. Scrape the flesh out using a fork for a noodle-like result.
- In a blender, put in the sauce ingredients. Puree.
- In a mixing bowl, put in the ingredients for the noodles. Pour the sauce over the noodles. Mix well. Serve.

#28 Cauliflower Grits and Shrimp

Serves: 2

Ingredients:

Shrimp:

- 3 tablespoons Cajun seasoning (no salt)
- 1 pound large shrimp (peeled and deveined)
- 2 tablespoons butter
- Salt

Cauliflower Grits:

- 1 large clove garlic (chopped)
- 1 bag (12 ounces) frozen cauliflower
- Salt
- 2 tablespoons butter

Instructions:

- In a steamer, put in the cauliflower and garlic. Steam until tender. (Do not discard the steaming water.)
- In a food processor, put in the steamed cauliflower, garlic, and butter. Process to your desired consistency. You can add some steaming water at a time and salt then process again until your desired consistency is achieved. Set aside.

- In a bowl, put in the Cajun seasoning. Coat the shrimp with the seasoning liberally. Season with salt.
- In a skillet over medium heat, melt the butter. Put in the shrimp. Cook until they all turned pink on all sides.
- Portion the cauliflower grits between 2 bowls. Put the cooked shrimp on top. Pour the sauce from the skillet on the bowls. Serve.

#29 Shrimp Garlic Zoodles
Serves: 2

Ingredients:

- 3/4 pounds medium shrimp (peeled and deveined)
- 2 medium zucchini
- 4 cloves garlic (minced)
- 1 tablespoon olive oil
- Red pepper flakes
- Zest and juice of 1 lemon
- Pepper
- Salt
- Fresh parsley (chopped)

Instructions:

- Using a spiralizer on medium setting, make the zoodles. Set aside.
- In a skillet over medium heat, put in the olive oil, zest, and lemon juice. Stir in the shrimp. Cook for a minute or two.
- Stir in the red pepper flakes and garlic. Cook for a minute more.
- Put in the zoodles. Toss for 3 minutes until slightly cooked.
- Season with pepper and salt. Garnish with parsley. Serve.

#30 Green Curry
Serves: 8

Ingredients:

- 3 cups broccoli florets
- 12 ounces tofu (firm)
- 3 cans (14 ounces) coconut milk
- 4 tablespoons green curry paste
- 2 sweet potatoes (peeled and cubed)
- A sprinkle of salt
- A swish of olive oil

Garnish:

- Golden raisins
- Fresh cilantro (chopped)
- Brown sugar
- Fish sauce

Instructions:

- Pat dry the tofu using paper towels. Slice the tofu into cubes.
- In a pot over medium heat, put in the olive oil. Put in the tofu. Season with salt. Fry the tofu for 15 minutes until all sides are golden brown. Set aside.
- In the same pot over medium heat, put in the coconut milk, sweet potatoes, and curry paste. Let simmer for 10 minutes. Put in the tofu and broccoli. Simmer for 5 minutes more.
- Garnish. Serve.

Chapter 8: Dinner Recipes

#1 Turkey Chili with Avocado
Serves: 8

Ingredients:

- 1 pound ground turkey
- 4 cups chicken broth
- 1 can (15 ounces) white beans
- 1 can (15 ounces) corn kernels
- 1 large white onion (diced)
- 1 avocado (diced)
- 4 garlic cloves (minced)
- 2 tablespoons extra-virgin olive oil
- 2 teaspoons ground cumin
- 1 teaspoon cayenne pepper
- 1 teaspoon ground coriander
- Salt
- Freshly ground black pepper

Instructions:

- In a pot over medium heat, put in the olive oil. Sautee the onion for 8 minutes. Stir in the garlic. Sautee for another minute.

- Put in the turkey. Cook for 7 minutes until cooked through. Put in the cayenne, coriander, cumin, salt, and pepper. Stir. Cook for a couple of minutes.
- Pour in the broth. Let the mixture simmer for 35 minutes over low heat.
- Put in the beans and corn. Simmer for 3 minutes more.
- Top each serving with diced avocado. Serve.

#2 Stir-Fried Snap Pea and Chicken
Serves: 4

Ingredients:

- 1 1/4 cups chicken breast (boneless, skinless, and sliced thinly)
- 2 1/2 cups snap peas
- 1 bunch scallions (sliced thinly)
- 1 red bell pepper (sliced thinly)
- 2 tablespoons vegetable oil
- 3 tablespoons fresh cilantro (chopped, + more for garnish)
- 3 tablespoons soy sauce
- 2 tablespoons sesame seeds (+ more for garnish)
- 2 tablespoons rice vinegar

- 2 teaspoons Sriracha
- 2 garlic cloves (minced)
- Freshly ground black pepper
- Salt

Instructions:

- In a pan over medium heat, put in the oil. Sautee the garlic and scallions for a minute. Stir in the snap peas and bell pepper. Sautee for 3 minutes.
- Put in the chicken. Cook for 5 minutes more.
- Put in the rice vinegar, soy sauce, sesame seeds, and Sriracha. Stir to combine. Simmer for 2 minutes.
- Put in the cilantro. Stir.
- Garnish each serving with sesame seeds and cilantro. Serve.

#3 Turkey Burgers with Tzatziki Sauce

Serves: 4 burgers

Ingredients:

Burgers:

- 1 pound ground turkey
- 1/2 cup fresh parsley (chopped)
- 3/4 cup bread crumbs

- 1 sweet onion (minced)
- 1 egg
- 2 garlic cloves (minced)
- 1 tablespoon extra-virgin olive oil
- 1/4 teaspoon red-pepper flakes
- 1/2 teaspoon dried oregano
- Freshly ground black pepper
- Salt

Tzatziki Sauce:

- 1/2 European cucumber (diced)
- 1 cup Greek yogurt
- 1/4 cup fresh parsley (chopped)
- 2 tablespoons lemon juice
- 1 tablespoon extra-virgin olive oil
- 1 pinch garlic powder
- Freshly ground black pepper
- Salt

Toppings:

- 8 Boston lettuce leaves
- 4 hamburger buns (whole-wheat)
- 2 tomatoes (sliced)
- 1/2 red onion (sliced)

Instructions:

Burgers:

- In a skillet over medium heat, put in the oil. Sautee the onion for 4 minutes. Put in the garlic. Sautee for another minute. Set aside.
- In a mixing bowl, put in the turkey, red pepper flakes, oregano, parsley, egg, and cooled onion. Mix well. Put in the bread crumbs, pepper, and salt. Mix well.
- Pre-heat your oven to 375 degrees Fahrenheit. Shape the turkey mixture into 4 patties.
- In an oven-safe skillet over medium heat, generously grease it with cooking spray.
- Put in the burger. Sear each side for 5 minutes until browned. Put the skillet in the oven. Bake the burgers for 17 minutes until cooked through.

Tzatziki Sauce:

- In a mixing bowl, put in the garlic powder, lemon juice, olive oil, cucumber, and yogurt. Mix well. Season with pepper and salt. Put in the parsley.

Toppings:

- Layer the burgers in this order: bun, 1/4 cup tzatziki sauce, two lettuce, two slices of tomato, and bun. Serve.

#4 Ratatouille

Yes, this is the same recipe as in the animated movie

Serves: 4

Ingredients:

- 1 cup tomato sauce
- 1 medium red onion (thickly sliced)
- 1 small eggplant (thickly sliced)
- 2 medium summer squash (thickly sliced)
- 2 small red bell peppers (halved)
- 2 medium zucchini (thickly sliced)
- 3 medium tomatoes (thickly sliced)
- 2 sprigs oregano
- 2 garlic cloves (smashed)
- 5 tablespoons olive oil
- 2 tablespoons thyme leaves
- Freshly ground black pepper
- Salt

Instructions:

- Preheat your oven to 375 degrees Fahrenheit. Arrange four small baking dishes on a baking sheet.
- In a pot over medium heat, put in the olive oil. Sautee the garlic for a minute. Turn off the heat. Stir in the oregano. Steep for 15 minutes. Discard the oregano and garlic.
- Grease each small baking dish with 2 teaspoons of the olive oil.
- Spread a couple of tablespoons of tomato sauce on each baking dish.
- Layer each baking dish with eggplant, onion, squash, zucchini, bell pepper, and tomato. Slightly stagger the slices and tightly packed.
- Spread the rest of the tomato sauce on top. Drizzle with the rest of the olive oil. Season with thyme, pepper, and salt.
- Roast for 30 minutes. Cool for a few minutes. Serve.

#5 Balsamic Chicken, Cranberries, Brussels Sprouts, and Pumpkin Seeds

Serves: 4

Ingredients:

- 1 1/4 pounds chicken breast (boneless, skinless, and bite-size slices)
- 20 Brussels sprouts (trimmed and halved)
- 1/2 cup dried cranberries
- 1/2 cup sun-dried tomatoes (dry)
- 1/2 cup roasted pumpkin seeds
- 1/4 cup balsamic vinegar
- 1 large shallot (peeled and diced)
- 3 tablespoons olive oil (divided)
- 2 tablespoons honey
- Pepper
- Salt

Instructions:

- In a skillet over medium heat, put in a couple tablespoons of olive oil. Arrange the Brussels sprouts with the cut side down. Sear them for 5 minutes.
- Pile the Brussels sprouts to one side of the skillet.
- Put in the rest of the olive oil on the empty surface of the skillet. Put in the shallots,

chicken, pepper, and salt. Cook for 5 minutes with constant stirring.
- Stir in the honey and balsamic vinegar. Lower the heat. Simmer for 3 minutes.
- Stir in the cranberries, tomatoes, and pumpkin seeds. Serve.

#6 Fried Rice with Pineapple
Serves: 4

Ingredients:

- 3 cups brown rice (cooked)
- 1/2 cup frozen corn
- 2 cups pineapple (diced)
- 1/2 cup frozen peas
- 1/2 cup ham (diced)
- 3 tablespoons soy sauce
- 2 tablespoons olive oil
- 1 tablespoon sesame oil
- 2 green onions (sliced)
- 2 carrots (peeled and grated)
- 1 onion (diced)
- 2 cloves garlic (minced)
- 1/4 teaspoon white pepper
- 1/2 teaspoon ginger powder

Instructions:

- In a bowl, put in the sesame oil, soy sauce, white pepper, and ginger powder. Mix well.
- In a skillet over medium heat, put in the olive oil. Sautee the onion and garlic for 4 minutes. Put in the peas, corn, and carrots. Cook for 4 minutes.
- Put in the rice, ham, pineapple, soy sauce mixture, and green onions. Cook for a couple of minutes with constant stirring. Serve.

#7 Baked Salmon with Sesame Seeds and Ginger in Parchment Packets
Serves: 4

Ingredients:

- 4 (6 ounces) salmon fillets (skinless)
- 2 large zucchini (halved lengthwise and sliced thinly)
- 1 lime (quartered)
- 1 red onion (halved and sliced thinly)
- 2 tablespoons soy sauce
- 2 tablespoons honey

- 2 tablespoons fresh ginger (grated)
- 4 teaspoons sesame seeds
- 1 teaspoon garlic powder
- 1 teaspoon sesame oil
- Pinch of red-pepper flakes

Instructions:

- Preheat your oven to 350 degrees Fahrenheit. Have four pieces of parchment paper ready.
- In a bowl, put in the ginger, soy sauce, honey, garlic powder, and red pepper flakes. Mix well.
- Make a parchment packet for each salmon fillet. Arrange 1/4 of the zucchini slices on a parchment paper. Top with 1/4 of the onion slices. Squeeze a lime segment on top.
- Put a salmon fillet on top. Brush generously with the soy sauce-honey mixture. Top with a teaspoon of sesame seeds.
- Fold the parchment paper carefully to seal the dish. Do the same process with the rest of the ingredients.
- Arrange the 4 parchment packets on a baking sheet. Bake for 18 minutes. Serve.

#8 Roasted Chicken with Fennel and Turmeric

Serves: 6

Ingredients:

- 1/2 cup dry white wine
- 1/2 cup extra virgin olive oil
- 1/2 cup orange juice
- 6 chicken breasts (bone in and skin on)
- 1 large fennel bulb (cored and sliced)
- 2 oranges (unpeeled and sliced)
- 1 large sweet onion (half moon slices)
- 1 lime (thinly sliced)
- 1 lime (juiced)
- 3 tablespoons brown sugar
- 2 tablespoons yellow mustard
- 3/4 tablespoon ground turmeric spice
- 1 tablespoon garlic powder
- 1 teaspoon sweet paprika
- 1 teaspoon ground coriander
- Pepper
- Salt

Instructions:

- In a mixing bowl, put in the brown sugar, mustard, lime juice, orange juice, white wine, and olive oil. Mix well the marinade.

- In another bowl, put in the paprika, pepper, coriander, salt, garlic powder, and turmeric. Mix well. Put half of the spice mixture into the marinade. Mix well.
- Pat dry the chicken breasts with paper towels. Season and coat well each chicken breast with the spice mixture.
- Put in the chicken breasts and the rest of the spice mixture into the marinade. Mix well. Marinate the chicken for 2 hours or more in the fridge.
- Pre-heat your oven to 475 degrees Fahrenheit. Put the chicken together with the marinade in a baking pan. Season with salt and brown sugar.
- Roast for 45 minutes. Serve.

#9 Eggs with Tomatoes and Asparagus

Serves: 4

Ingredients:

- 1 pint cherry tomatoes
- 2 pounds asparagus
- 4 eggs
- 2 teaspoons fresh thyme (chopped)
- 2 tablespoons olive oil

- Pepper
- Salt

Instructions:

- Pre-heat your oven to 400 degrees Fahrenheit. Grease a baking pan with cooking spray.
- Put the tomatoes and asparagus in a single layer on the greased baking pan. Drizzle with the olive oil. Season with pepper, salt, and thyme.
- Roast for 12 minutes. Remove from the oven.
- Crack the eggs over the asparagus. Season with pepper and salt.
- Bake for 7 minutes. Serve.

#10 Bulgur and Sweet Potato Salad

Serves: 4

Ingredients:

- 2 medium sweet potatoes (peeled and diced)
- 1 1/4 cups bulgur wheat
- 1 cup parsley (finely chopped)
- 1/2 cup mint (finely chopped)
- 1/4 cup olive oil

- 1/4 cup red onion (finely chopped)
- 1/4 cup orange juice (freshly squeezed)
- 2 tablespoons orange zest
- 2 tablespoons lemon juice
- 1 tablespoon red wine vinegar
- 1 tablespoon avocado oil
- 2 teaspoons maple syrup
- 1/2 teaspoon salt
- 1 small clove garlic (grated)
- Coarse salt
- Black pepper
- Freshly ground black pepper

Instructions:

- Pre-heat your oven to 425 degrees Fahrenheit. Line a baking sheet with parchment paper.
- In a bowl, put in the sweet potatoes, avocado oil, and maple syrup. Season with salt and pepper. Toss to combine.
- Spread evenly on the lined baking sheet. Roast for 40 minutes. Stir halfway through the roasting.
- In a pot over medium heat, put in 3 1/2 cups water. Bring to a boil. Put in the bulgur. Stir. Lower the heat. Simmer for 8 minutes with occasional stirring. Turn off the heat. Cover the pot. Let it sit for 10

minutes. Drain the liquid. Fluff the bulgur.
- In a bowl, put in the garlic, vinegar, pepper, salt, lemon juice, orange juice, and olive oil. Mix well.
- In another bowl, put in the bulgur, mint, parsley, orange zest, red onion, and the vinegar-garlic mixture. Toss to combine. Serve.

#11 Carrot, Turmeric, and Ginger Soup

Serves: 4

Ingredients:

- 4 cups vegetable stock
- 3 carrots (diced)
- 3 cloves garlic (minced)
- 1 white onion (diced)
- 1 inch fresh ginger (finely grated)
- 1 tablespoon lemon juice
- 2 inches fresh turmeric (finely grated)
- Black sesame seeds (for topping)
- Canned coconut milk (for topping)

Instructions:

- In a pot over medium heat, put in some olive oil. Sautee the onion until soft. Put in the garlic, ginger, and turmeric. Sautee for 1 more minute.
- Put in the carrots. Cook for 2 minutes. Put in the vegetable stock. Simmer for 25 minutes.
- Blend the soup using a stick blender. Put in the lemon juice. Stir. Serve with black sesame seeds and a swirl of coconut milk.

#12 Salmon Roast with Romaine and Potatoes

Serves: 4

Ingredients:

- 1 pound baby potatoes (rinsed)
- 2 hearts romaine lettuce (cut in half)
- 4 (6-ounce) salmon fillets
- 4 tablespoons olive oil (divided)
- 1 tablespoon butter (melted)
- 1 teaspoon lemon juice
- 1/4 teaspoon paprika
- Freshly ground black pepper
- Salt

Instructions:

- Pre-heat your oven to 400 degrees Fahrenheit. Grease a baking tray with cooking spray.
- In a bowl, put in the half of the olive oil and potatoes. Toss to coat. Spread out the potatoes on the greased baking tray.
- Roast for 20 minutes.
- Rub the romaine lettuce with lemon juice and the other half of the olive oil. Season with pepper and salt.
- Brush the melted butter on the salmon fillets. Season with pepper, salt, and paprika.
- Arrange the salmon fillets and romaine lettuce on the baking tray with the potatoes. Roast for another 7 minutes. Serve.

#13 Peppers Stuffed with Sweet Potato and Turkey

Serves: 4

Ingredients:

- 2 cups ground turkey
- 1 2/3 cups sweet potatoes (diced)
- 1/2 cup tomato sauce
- 1/2 cup onions (diced)
- 2 large bell peppers (cut in half)
- 1 tablespoon extra virgin olive oil
- 2 cloves garlic (minced)
- Pepper
- Salt
- Fresh parsley (for garnishing)

Instructions:

- Pre-heat your oven to 350 degrees Fahrenheit. Grease a baking tray with cooking spray.
- In a skillet over medium heat, put in the olive oil. Put in the garlic and turkey. Cook for 10 minutes with occasional stirring to break up the meat.
- Put in the onions. Cook for 5 minutes.
- Stir in the potatoes. Cover. Cook for 8 minutes with occasional stirring.
- Put in the tomato sauce, pepper, and salt.

- Arrange the bell peppers on the greased baking tray. The cavity is facing up.
- Fill each bell pepper to the brim with the sweet potato-turkey mixture.
- Bake for 30 minutes.
- Garnish with parsley. Serve.

#14 Bean Bolognese
Serves: 4

Ingredients:

- 1 can (28-ounce) crushed tomatoes
- 1 can (14-ounce) white beans
- 1 medium onion (chopped)
- 2 celery stalks (chopped)
- 2 carrots (peeled and chopped)
- 2 cloves garlic (minced)

Instructions:

- In a crock pot, put in all the ingredients. Cook for 6 hours. Serve.

#15 Turkey Meatballs

Serves: 30 mini balls

Ingredients:

- 1 pound ground turkey
- 1/2 cup fresh Parmesan cheese (grated)
- 1/2 cup fresh breadcrumbs (whole wheat)
- 1 large egg (beaten)
- 2-3 tablespoons water
- 1 tablespoon fresh parsley (chopped)
- 1/2 tablespoon fresh oregano (chopped)
- 1/2 tablespoon fresh basil (chopped)
- Pinch of fresh nutmeg (grated)

Instructions:

- Pre-heat your oven to 350 degrees Fahrenheit. Line two baking trays with parchment paper.
- In a mixing bowl, put in the turkey, cheese, breadcrumbs, egg, herbs, water, nutmeg, pepper, and salt. Mix well. Add more water if the mixture is not sticky enough to form into a ball.
- Shape the mixture into 30 mini balls. Arrange the balls on the lined baking trays.
- Bake for 30 minutes. Turn the balls halfway through the baking. Serve.

#16 Cauliflower Rice and Salmon Bowl

Serves: 2

Ingredients:

- 2 salmon fillets
- 1/2 head cauliflower (riced)
- 1 bunch kale (shredded)
- 12 Brussels sprouts (halved)
- 3 tablespoons olive oil
- Himalayan salt
- 1 teaspoon curry powder

Marinade:

- 1/4 cup tamari sauce
- 1 tablespoon sesame seeds
- 1 teaspoon Dijon mustard
- 1 teaspoon maple syrup
- 1 teaspoon sesame oil

Instructions:

- Pre-heat your oven to 350 degrees Fahrenheit. Line a baking sheet with parchment paper.
- Put the Brussels sprouts on the lined baking sheet. Coat with a tablespoon of olive oil. Season with salt. Roast for 20 minutes.

- In a bowl, put in all the ingredients for the marinade. Mix well.
- Replace the Brussels sprouts with the salmon fillets on the baking sheet. Coat the fillets with the marinade. Bake for 15 minutes.
- In a pan over medium heat, put in a tablespoon of olive oil. Sautee the kale for 3 minutes. Set aside.
- In the same pan over medium heat, put in the rest of the olive oil. Put in the cauliflower rice, curry powder, and salt. Sautee for 3 minutes.
- Portion the Brussels sprouts and salmon fillets between two bowls. Top with cauliflower rice and kale. Serve.

#17 Chicken Chili and White Beans

Serves: 6

Ingredients:

- 3 cups chicken stock
- 2 cups cooked chicken breast (shredded)
- 1 cup Brussels sprouts (chopped)
- 1 cup nut milk
- 1 can (15-ounce) small white beans
- 2 tablespoons olive oil
- 1 tablespoon ground cumin
- 1 leek (chopped)
- 1 small onion (chopped)
- 2 garlic cloves (minced)
- 1 jalapeño pepper (seeded and diced)
- 1 teaspoon dried oregano
- 1 large white potato (peeled and chopped)
- Pinch of crushed red pepper flakes

Garnish:

- Shredded cheese
- Jalapeño slices
- Hot sauce
- Tortilla chips

Instructions:

- In a pot over medium heat, put in the olive oil. Sautee the leek, onion, and jalapeño for 5 minutes.
- Stir in the spices and garlic. Cook for a minute.
- Put the Brussels sprouts, potato, white beans, stock, and chicken. Stir. Simmer for 20 minutes.
- Put in the milk. Stir. Cook for a minute. Serve with the garnishes.

#18 Harissa and Chicken Tenders
Serves: 6

Ingredients:

- 24 pieces chicken tenders (boneless and skinless)
- 2 tablespoons harissa paste
- 1/4 cup dry white wine
- 1/4 cup plain Greek yogurt

Instructions:

- In a bowl, put in the yogurt, harissa, and wine. Mix well.
- Put in the chicken tenders. Coat the tenders with the marinade. Cover.

- Marinate in the fridge for 2 hours or more.
- Heat up your grill. Drain the chicken tenders. Let the excess liquid drip off. Grill the tenders for 5 minutes per side.
- Serve the tenders in a sandwich. Top with fresh herbs and vegetable slices of your choice.

#19 Baked Cauliflower Buffalo

Serves: 4

Ingredients:

- 1/2 cup hot sauce
- 1/4 cup water
- 1/4 cup banana flour
- 1 medium cauliflower (bite-sized)
- 2 tablespoons butter (melted)
- Pinch of pepper
- Pinch of salt
- Ranch dressing (for serving)

Instructions:

- Preheat your oven to 425 degrees Fahrenheit. Line a baking sheet with foil.
- In a mixing bowl, put in the water, flour, pepper, and salt. Mix well.

- Put in the cauliflower. Toss to coat well. Spread out the coated cauliflower on the lined baking sheet.
- Bake for 15 minutes. Flip the cauliflower halfway through the baking.
- In another bowl, put in the hot sauce and butter. Mix well. Drizzle the mixture over the cauliflower. Bake again for another 20 minutes. Serve with the ranch dressing.

#20 Chinese Chicken Salad

Serves: 4

Ingredients:

Dressing:

- 1/2 cup vegetable oil
- 1/4-inch ginger (peeled and chopped)
- 1/4 cup rice wine vinegar (unseasoned)
- 1 tablespoon soy sauce (low-sodium)
- 1 tablespoon Dijon mustard
- 2 garlic cloves (minced)
- 1 teaspoon sesame oil
- Pinch of salt

Salad:

- 4 cups green cabbage (shredded)

- 1/4 cup cooked edamame
- 1 cup red cabbage (shredded)
- 1/2 cup cilantro leaves (chopped)
- 2 cooked chicken breasts (shredded)
- 1 small carrot (thin strips)
- 4 scallions (thinly sliced)
- 2 tablespoons mint leaves (chopped)
- Wonton strips

Instructions:

- In a blender, put in all the dressing ingredients. Pulse until smooth in texture.
- In a mixing bowl, put in all the salad ingredients. Pour the dressing over the salad. Toss to mix well. Garnish with wonton strips. Serve.

#21 Kale and Sweet Potato Tostadas

Serves: 4

Ingredients:

- 8 stems kale (roughly chopped)
- 2 medium sweet potatoes (cleaned and chopped)
- 12 Brussels sprouts (finely chopped)
- 2 tablespoons olive oil
- 1 tablespoon lime juice
- 1 tablespoon olive oil
- 1 teaspoon honey
- Pinch of salt
- Pinch of cayenne pepper
- Corn tortillas
- Toasted coconut
- Yogurt
- Fresh mint (chopped)

Instructions:

- Pre-heat your oven to 400 degrees Fahrenheit. Line two baking sheets with foil.
- Put the sweet potatoes on one lined baking sheet. Drizzle with olive oil. Season with cayenne pepper. Toss to coat.

- Put the kale on the other lined baking sheet. Drizzle with olive oil. Season with salt. Toss to coat.
- Put both baking sheets in the oven. Roast the kale for 10 minutes only. Roast the sweet potatoes for 40 minutes.
- In a bowl, put in the honey, lime juice, and Brussels sprouts. Toss to coat well.
- Put as many corn tortillas as you want on a tin foil. Put it inside the warm oven for 3 minutes to get toasted.
- Layer the sweet potatoes and kale on a tortilla. Top with the Brussels sprouts, yogurt, mint, and toasted coconut. Serve.

#22 Saag Paneer
Serves: 4

Ingredients:

- 20 ounces frozen spinach (finely chopped)
- 8 ounces paneer cheese (1/2-inch cubes)
- 2 cups low-fat plain yogurt
- 1 jalapeño pepper (finely chopped)
- 1 small onion (finely chopped)
- 1 clove garlic (minced)
- 2 tablespoons extra-virgin olive oil (divided)

- 2 teaspoons garam masala
- 1 tablespoon fresh ginger (minced)
- 1 teaspoon ground cumin
- 1/4 teaspoon ground turmeric
- 3/4 teaspoon salt

Instructions:

- In a bowl, put in the turmeric and paneer. Toss to coat well.
- In a skillet over medium heat, put in a tablespoon of olive oil. Put in the paneer. Cook for 5 minutes with occasional flipping to brown all sides. Set aside.
- In the same skillet over medium heat, put in the remaining olive oil. Sautee the jalapeño and onion for 8 minutes. Add 2 tablespoons of water at a time if the pan is dry when cooking.
- Stir in the cumin, ginger, garlic, and garam masala. Cook for less than a minute.
- Stir in the spinach and salt. Cook for 3 minutes. Turn off the heat.
- Stir in the paneer and yogurt. Serve.

#23 Green Fried Rice
Serves: 4

Ingredients:

- 2 cups brown rice (cooked)
- 1/2 cup broccoli (chopped)
- 1/2 cup peas (frozen or fresh)
- 1 celery stalk (diced)
- 1 garlic clove (minced)
- 1 small white onion (diced)
- 1 tablespoon olive oil
- 1 tablespoon tamari sauce
- 1/4 teaspoon fresh lemon zest
- 1 teaspoon honey

Instructions:

- In a pan over medium heat, put in the olive oil. Sautee the onion, broccoli, and celery for 2 minutes.
- Put in the rice and garlic. Cook for 2 minutes more.
- Put in the honey, tamari, and peas. Cook for another 5 minutes with regular stirring.
- Turn off the heat. Put in the lemon zest. Mix well. Serve.

#24 Baked Tilapia with Rosemary
Serves: 4

Ingredients:

- 4 (4 ounces) tilapia fillets
- 1/3 cup whole wheat panko breadcrumbs
- 1/3 cup raw pecans (chopped)
- 1 egg white
- 2 teaspoons fresh rosemary (chopped)
- 1 1/2 teaspoon olive oil
- 1/8 teaspoon salt
- 1/2 teaspoon brown sugar
- 1 pinch cayenne pepper

Instructions:

- Pre-heat your oven to 350 degrees Fahrenheit.
- In a baking dish, put in the cayenne pepper, salt, sugar, rosemary, breadcrumbs, and pecans. Mix well. Put in the olive oil. Toss to coat.
- Bake for 8 minutes. Set aside.
- Change the oven temperature to 400 degrees Fahrenheit. Grease a glass baking dish with cooking spray.
- Whisk the egg white in a shallow dish.
- Dip a tilapia fillet into the egg white. Coat the fillet well with the pecan mixture. Put

the coated fillet in the greased baking dish. Do this step with the rest of the tilapia fillets.
- Coat the top of the tilapia fillets with the remaining pecan mixture.
- Bake for 10 minutes. Serve.

#25 Chickpea and Sweet Potato Stew

Serves: 6

Ingredients:

- 2 medium sweet potatoes (peeled and diced)
- 1 cup vegetable stock
- 1 can (14-ounce) coconut milk
- 2 cans (14-ounce) chickpeas
- 2 garlic cloves (minced)
- 2 carrots (chopped)
- 1 small white onion (chopped)
- 1-inch ginger (minced)
- 2 tablespoons olive oil
- 1 teaspoon paprika
- 1 teaspoon cumin
- 1/4 teaspoon ground turmeric
- Pinch of pepper
- Pinch of salt

Instructions:

- In a pot over medium heat, put in the olive oil. Sautee the onion and carrots for 10 minutes.
- Stir in the spices, ginger, and garlic. Cook for a minute more.
- Put in the rest of the ingredients. Bring to a boil. Cover the pot. Lower the heat. Simmer for 1 hour. Serve.

#26 Winter Squash and Tofu Lasagna
Serves: 6

Ingredients:

- 1-pound lasagna noodles (no-boil)
- 4 cups prepared Marinara sauce
- 2 cups winter squash (cooked and mashed)
- 1/2 cup coconut milk
- 1 package (16-ounce) soft tofu
- 2 tablespoons fresh lemon juice
- 1 tablespoon packed brown sugar
- 1 tablespoon fresh thyme leaves
- Salt
- Pinch smoked paprika

- Pepper

Instructions:

- Pre-heat your oven to 350 degrees Fahrenheit.
- In a mixing bowl, put in the brown sugar and squash. Mix well.
- In a food processor, put in the paprika, thyme, lemon juice, and tofu. Process until smooth.
- Pour the tofu mixture into squash. Season with pepper and salt. Combine well.
- Spread a thin layer of Marinara sauce on the bottom of a baking dish (9" x 13"). Layer the noodles on top (a third of the package). Next is a layer of the tofu-squash mixture (a third of the mixture).
- Continue layering in this order: Marinara sauce, noodles, and tofu-squash mixture.
- Bake for 45 minutes. Serve.

#27 Rosemary-Walnut Crusted Salmon

Serves: 4

Ingredients:

- 1 pound skinless salmon fillet
- 3 tablespoons walnuts (finely chopped)
- 3 tablespoons panko breadcrumbs
- 1 clove garlic (minced)
- 2 teaspoons Dijon mustard
- 1 teaspoon extra-virgin olive oil
- 1 teaspoon fresh rosemary (chopped)
- 1 teaspoon lemon juice
- 1/2 teaspoon kosher salt
- 1/2 teaspoon honey
- 1/4 teaspoon crushed red pepper
- 1/4 teaspoon lemon zest
- Olive oil cooking spray
- Lemon wedges (for garnish)
- Fresh parsley (chopped)

Instructions:

- Pre-heat your oven to 425 degrees Fahrenheit. Line a rimmed baking tray with parchment paper.
- In a bowl, put in the crushed red pepper, salt, honey, rosemary, lemon juice, lemon zest, garlic, and mustard. Mix well.

- In another bowl, put in the oil, walnuts, and breadcrumbs. Mix well.
- Put the salmon on the lined baking tray. Spread the rosemary mixture on top of the fish. Press the breadcrumb mixture over the fish to adhere. Coat lightly with the cooking spray.
- Bake for 12 minutes. Garnish with lemon wedges and parsley. Serve.

#28 Maple Miso Salmon
Serves: 8

Ingredients:

- 2 1/2 pound salmon fillet (skin-on)
- 2 limes
- 2 lemons
- 1/4 cup white miso
- 2 tablespoons maple syrup
- 2 tablespoons extra-virgin olive oil
- 1/4 teaspoon ground pepper
- Sliced scallions (for garnish)
- Pinch of cayenne pepper

Instructions:

- Place a rack in the upper third of your oven. Pre-heat your oven to broiler-high. Line a rimmed baking tray with foil.
- In a bowl, juice a lime and a lemon. Put in the miso, pepper, oil, cayenne, and maple syrup. Mix well.
- Put the salmon on the lined baking tray, the skin-side down. Slice in half the last lemon and lime. Put them around the salmon, the cut-sides up.
- Broil for 12 minutes. Garnish with scallions. Serve.

#29 Cauliflower and Broccoli Salad
Serves: 6

Ingredients:

- 8 cups lacinato kale (chopped)
- 3 cups broccoli florets
- 3 cups cauliflower florets
- 1 cup manchego cheese (shaved)
- 1/2 cup dried cherries
- 1/3 cup toasted pecans (chopped)
- 4 tablespoons extra-virgin olive oil (divided)
- 1 tablespoon champagne vinegar

- 1 1/2 teaspoons Dijon mustard
- 1/2 teaspoon salt (divided)
- 1 teaspoon honey
- 1/4 teaspoon ground pepper

Instructions:

- Position a rimmed baking tray in the middle rack of your oven. Pre-heat to 450 degrees Fahrenheit.
- In a bowl, put in the broccoli and cauliflower. Mix well.
- Put in the pepper, half of the salt, and half of the olive oil. Toss to coat the vegetables.
- Put on the pre-heated baking tray. Roast for 12 minutes, turning once.
- In another bowl, put in the rest of the salt, rest of the olive oil, honey, mustard, and vinegar. Mix well.
- Put in the kale. Massage the dressing into the kale for 3 minutes with your hands.
- Put in the roasted vegetables, cheese, cherries, and pecans. Toss well. Serve.

#30 Watercress, Raspberry, and Peach Salad with Five-Spice Bacon

Serves: 4

Ingredients:

Five-Spice Bacon:

- 8 ounces bacon (thick-cut)
- 1/4 cup red wine
- 1/4 cup port
- 1 tablespoon pure maple syrup
- 1 1/2 teaspoons Chinese five-spice powder
- 2 cloves garlic (peeled)

Salad:

- 4 cups watercress (trimmed)
- 3/4 cup fresh raspberries
- 3 firm ripe peaches (1/4-inch wedges)
- 1 medium shallot (thinly sliced)
- 1/2 small head radicchio (separate leaves and cut into 1-inch strips)
- 2 tablespoons cider vinegar
- 2 tablespoons extra-virgin olive oil
- 1/4 teaspoon Chinese five-spice powder
- 1 teaspoon pure maple syrup
- Pinch of sea salt

Instructions:

Five-Spice Bacon:

- Slice the bacon into strips (1/4-inch thick).
- In a skillet over medium heat, put the bacon. Cook for 5 minutes with constant stirring.
- Place the bacon on paper towels to absorb the excess grease. Throw away the grease left on the skillet.
- In the same skillet over high heat, put in the five-spice powder, garlic, maple syrup, wine, and port. Bring to a boil.
- Put in the bacon. Cook for 2 1/2 minutes with constant stirring. Turn off the heat.

Salad:

- In a bowl, put in the five-spice powder, maple syrup, olive oil, vinegar, salt, and shallot. Mix well.
- Put in the raspberries. Crush them lightly when mixing.
- Put in the watercress, peaches, and radicchio. Toss well.
- Top each salad serving with the bacon.

Chapter 8: Snack Recipes

#1 Turmeric Gummies
Serves: 4

Ingredients:

- 3 1/2 cups water
- 8 tablespoons gelatin powder (unflavored)
- 6 tablespoons maple syrup
- 1 teaspoon ground turmeric
- Pinch of ground pepper

Instructions:

- In a pot, over medium heat, put in the water, maple syrup, and turmeric. Cook for 5 minutes with stirring.
- Turn off the heat. Stir in the gelatin powder. Mix well.
- Turn on the heat. Mix well the mixture in the pot to dissolve the gelatin powder.
- Pour the mixture into silicon molds. Cover. Chill in the fridge for 4 hours or more to become firm.
- Slice into bite-size gummies. Serve.

#2 Spicy Tuna Rolls

Serves: 6 rolls

Ingredients:

- 1 pouch Yellowfin Tuna
- 1 medium cucumber
- 2 avocado slices (cut into 6 pieces in total)
- 1 teaspoon hot sauce
- 1/8 teaspoon pepper
- 1/8 teaspoon salt
- 1/16 teaspoon ground cayenne

Instructions:

- Thinly slice the cucumber lengthwise. There should be no seeds in the slice cucumbers. Make a total of 6 slices. Pat dry the slices with paper towels.
- In a mixing bowl, put in the tuna, cayenne, pepper, salt, and hot sauce. Mix well.
- Spread the tuna mixture on the cucumber slices. Leave some space on the sides.
- Put an avocado piece on the top. Roll the cucumber carefully. Secure each roll with toothpicks. Serve.

#3 Ginger-Cinnamon Mixed Nuts
Serves: 8

Ingredients:

- 2 cups mixed nuts
- 2 large egg whites
- 1 teaspoon fresh ginger (grated)
- 1/2 teaspoon ground Vietnamese cinnamon
- 1/2 teaspoon fine sea salt
- Coconut oil spray

Instructions:

- Pre-heat your oven to 250 degrees Fahrenheit.
- In a mixing bowl, put the egg whites. Whip until frothy.
- Put in the cinnamon, salt, and ginger. Whip until well combined.
- Put in the mixed nuts. Mix well to coat.
- Grease a parchment paper with coconut oil spray. Put the parchment paper on a baking sheet. Spread the nuts in a single layer on the parchment paper.
- Bake for 40 minutes. Rotate the baking sheet halfway through.
- Let the nuts cool down and harden. Break them into pieces. Serve.

#4 Spicy Kale Chips

Serves: 4

Ingredients:

- 1 bunch of curly kale (rinsed and pat dried)
- 1/4 teaspoon ground cayenne pepper
- 1/4 teaspoon sea salt
- 1/8 teaspoon garlic powder
- 1/8 teaspoon black pepper
- Coconut oil spray

Instructions:

- Pre-heat your oven to 300 degrees Fahrenheit.
- Tear the kale leaves into the size of chips.
- Arrange the leaves on a baking wire rack, evenly spaced from each other. Put the rack on top of a cookie sheet lined with foil.
- Spray the leaves lightly with coconut oil.
- Season with cayenne pepper, garlic powder, and salt.
- Bake on the middle rack for 20 minutes. Serve.

#5 Ginger Date Almond Bars

Serves: 8 bars

Ingredients:

- 1 cup almond flour
- 1/4 cup almond milk
- 3/4 cup dates
- 1 teaspoon ground ginger

Instructions:

- Pre-heat your oven to 350 degrees Fahrenheit.
- In a blender, put in the almond milk and dates. Blend for 5 minutes to make a paste.
- Put in the ginger and almond flour. Blend for another 3 minutes.
- Put the mixture in a baking dish. Bake for 20 minutes.
- Let it cool. Slice into 8 bars. Serve.

#6 Turmeric Vanilla Orange Juice

Serves: 2

Ingredients:

- 1 cup almond milk (unsweetened)
- 3 oranges (peeled and quartered)
- 1 teaspoon vanilla extract
- 1/4 teaspoon turmeric
- 1/2 teaspoon cinnamon
- Pinch of pepper

Instructions:

- In a blender, put in all the ingredients.
- Blend until smooth. Serve.

#7 Baked Turmeric Veggie Nuggets

Serves: 24 nuggets

Ingredients:

- 2 cups broccoli florets
- 2 cups cauliflower florets
- 1 cup carrots (coarsely chopped)
- 1/2 cup almond meal
- 1 teaspoon garlic (minced)
- 1 large egg
- 1/2 teaspoon ground turmeric

- 1/4 teaspoon black pepper
- 1/4 teaspoon sea salt

Instructions:

- Pre-heat your oven to 400 degrees Fahrenheit. Line a baking tray with parchment paper.
- In a food processor, put in the cauliflower, broccoli, turmeric, carrots, salt, garlic, and pepper. Pulse until fine in texture.
- Put in the egg and almond meal. Pulse to mix.
- Pour into a mixing bowl. Shape the mixture into 24 nuggets. Arrange on the lined baking tray.
- Bake for 25 minutes, flipping halfway through the time. Serve.

#8 Energy Bites with Turmeric

Serves: 18 bites

Ingredients:

- 1 cup almond butter
- 6 tablespoons plant based protein powder
- 3/4 cup coconut flakes (unsweetened)
- 1 teaspoon coconut oil
- 2 teaspoons turmeric

- 1/2 teaspoon maple syrup

Instructions:

- In a blender, put in the butter, half of the coconut flakes, maple syrup, coconut oil, turmeric, and protein powder. Blend until mixed well.
- Spread the dough on a baking sheet. Refrigerate for an hour to become firm.
- Roll the dough into 18 bites. Arrange the bites on the baking sheet. Put in the fridge for 4 hours to harden.
- Roll each bite into the remaining coconut flakes. Serve.

#9 Ginger and Turmeric Smoothie

Serves: 1

Ingredients:

- 1 1/2 cups coconut milk (unsweetened)
- 1 cup ice
- 2 tablespoons pure honey
- 1 teaspoon coconut oil (softened)
- 1 teaspoon turmeric
- 1 teaspoon chia seeds
- 1 teaspoon ginger (peeled and chopped)

Instructions:

- In a blender, put in the ice, turmeric, coconut milk, honey, coconut oil, and ginger. Blend until smooth.
- Put in a glass. Stir in the chia seeds. Let the chia seeds bloom before serving.

#10 Coffee Cacao Protein Bars

Serves: 12 bars

Ingredients:

- 2 cups mixed nuts
- 18 large Medjool dates (pitted)
- 1 cup egg white protein powder
- 1/4 cup cacao nibs
- 1/4 cup cacao powder
- 5 tablespoons water
- 3 tablespoons instant coffee powder

Instructions:

- Line a square pan (8" x 8") with parchment paper.
- In a food processor, put in the nuts, cacao powder, egg white protein, and coffee. Process until the nuts are broken into small pieces only.

- Put in the dates. Process to combine. Pour a tablespoon of water at a time while processing until the mixture becomes sticky.
- Remove the S-blade of the processor. Stir in the cacao nibs into the mixture.
- Pour into the lined square pan. Flatten the mixture evenly using a roller.
- Put in the fridge for an hour. Slice into 16 bars. Serve.

Chapter 9: Seven-Day Meal Plan

The following is a seven-day meal plan that you can use to try the anti-inflammatory diet for an entire week. If you think it is something that is absolutely doable for you then you can create your own meal plan for the following weeks using the recipes found in the previous chapters.

If you want to see the recipes you just tap the name of the recipe.

Day 1

Breakfast: Scrambled Eggs with Turmeric

Lunch: Avocado Chickpea Salad Sandwich

Dinner: Turkey Chili with Avocado

Day 2

Breakfast: Chia Seed and Milk Pudding

Lunch: Buddha Bowl with Avocado, Kale, Wild Rice, and Orange

Dinner: Stir-Fried Snap Pea and Chicken

Day 3

Breakfast: Protein-Rich Turmeric Donuts

Lunch: Spiced Lentil Soup

Dinner: Turkey Burgers with Tzatziki Sauce

Day 4

Breakfast: Nutty Choco-Nana Pancakes

Lunch: Tuna Mediterranean Salad

Dinner: Ratatouille

Day 5

Breakfast: Cranberry and Sweet Potato Bars

Lunch: Red Lentil Pasta with Tomato

Dinner: Balsamic Chicken, Cranberries, Brussels Sprouts, and Pumpkin Seeds

Day 6

Breakfast: Turmeric Scones

Lunch: Chicken and Greek Salad Wrap

Dinner: Fried Rice with Pineapple

Day 7

Breakfast: Blueberry Avocado Chocolate Muffins

Lunch: Butternut Squash Carrot Soup

Dinner: Baked Salmon with Sesame Seeds and Ginger in Parchment Packets

For snack options, you can have any of the snacks provided in the sample recipes chapters. Alternatively, you can also snack on other anti-inflammatory food options from the shopping list that you can find in chapter 3 of this book.

Conclusion

Thank you again for purchasing and traversing this book from start to finish. It is my hope that the information provided here, the recipes, and meal plans have been very helpful to you.

Remember that this is only a beginner's introductory guide to the anti-inflammatory diet. As you keep to this diet you will reap the benefits such as better health, more manageable blood pressure, and reduced inflammation among other things.

I hope that you enjoyed the recipes as much as I enjoyed them when I first had them. I understand that switching to this diet may be difficult for some. But I promise you that you will live healthier and eat healthier with this type of diet.

To your health!